TEST TUBE BABIES
BABIES
– a Christian view

Papers from the Conference 'In Vitro Fertilisation and the Quality of Life' organised by the Order of Christian Unity at the Royal Society of Medicine, London, 23 May 1983

Foreword by
Sir John Peel
KCVO, DM, FRCOG, FRCP, FRCS, Hon FACOG

Unity Press
Becket Publications

© Order of Christian Unity 1984.
First published 1984 by Becket Publications, St. Thomas House, Oxford,
OX1 1SJ and Unity Press, London.

This Second Edition published 1985

ISBN 0 7289 0020 3

Printed in Great Britain by
Biddles Limited, Guildford.

FOREWORD

We are living in an era in which scientific and technological developments have exploded in such a dramatic way that it has become possible to do a great many things before society at large has had the time and opportunity to reflect and decide whether they should of necessity always be done. We can manufacture an atomic bomb but who would argue that it should be used?

In vitro fertilisation has been developed by a combination of scientific laboratory research and advanced technology applied to clinical practice. Its application to relieve infertility caused primarily by blockage of the fallopian tubes in the female, albeit that blockage has so often been caused by the patient's own prior fault, has nevertheless already brought untold happiness and relief to scores of childless couples and will continue to do so with greater frequency in the future. Furthermore it can have an application in cases where the risk is great that a child conceived in the normal way will become the victim of a disease or disorder due to some transmissible genetic defect. This involves the process of egg donation, similar in essence to A.I.D. which has been widely practised for many years. I.V.F. is not a panacea for all types of infertility but by any count it must be regarded as a wonderful medical achievement for those cases where it is indicated.

Why then should there be a concern about it? The reasons are many and varied and the reader of this booklet will find them enumerated and discussed in detail in a series of papers written by men and women of great distinction in their various professions, of the highest integrity and who are able to speak from a very wide range of experience. The issues involved are fundamental in their concern with the moral and ethical aspects of human reproduction. It is not therefore a matter solely for doctors in their clinical practice. If we believe, as we must do on purely scientific grounds alone, that life begins at conception (fertilisation), then the fertilised ovum is human and so entitled to all the protection that flows from a belief in the sanctity of human life. What is the status then of an in vitro conceptus? Now a whole range of possibilities are open to it – freezing – storing – experimenting – cloning – donation to a surrogate mother – implantation in the womb of an unmarried woman – and who knows what else in the future, perhaps even grown-on in an artificial environment until someone decides to kill it. This is not just science fiction but fact.

Anyone who claims to know all the answers to these very serious dilemmas would indeed be arrogant in the extreme. But the Order of Christian Unity, which organised the conference from which the papers in this booklet were subsequently prepared, believes firmly that a Christian viewpoint should be heard alongside all the other views that are being expressed. Marriage and the unity of family life are being steadily undermined and it would be tragic if a new medical technique which is capable of contributing greatly to both, were to fall into any disrepute because of abuse. The pages of this booklet will highlight all those dangers and I hope they will be very widely read. The origins of medicine were in religion and philosophy rather than in science, but for many years now medicine has become more allied to the latter rather than the former. The pages of this booklet will, I hope, focus the reader's mind on the view, held firmly by the Order of Christian Unity, that both religion and philosophy should still have an important influence on the practice of medicine.

CONTENTS

ACKNOWLEDGEMENTS

The success of the Conference on 'In Vitro Fertilisation and the Quality of Life' at the Royal Society of Medicine on 23 May 1983 was attributable to many factors. First, we were convinced that the hand of the Lord was on the Order of Christian Unity's initiative in calling the Conference in the first place. Then there was the hard working Committee chaired by Dr Chandra Sethurajan, Chairman of the OCU Medical Ethics Committee, and various officers and voluntary workers of the OCU. The distinguished panel of speakers, under the joint chairmanship of Professor Ian Donald and Sir John Peel deserve our especial thanks as it is their papers which are now reproduced here in book form: Professor James Scott, Dr David White, Mr Gerard Wright QC, Mr Rex Brinkworth, Dr Teresa Iglesias and our guest speaker from the University of Paris, Professor Jerome Lejeune. We wish also to acknowledge particularly the special contribution made by Lady Lothian, President, and Lady Watherston, Chairman of the OCU and all those who have assisted in the preparation of the texts and design of this book as well as those who have contributed to the Christian view of IVF which is reflected in this work.

In this Second Edition we acknowledge the contribution of the MORI Poll *In Vitro Fertilisation — A Survey of Public Attitudes*, July 1984, conducted for the Order of Christian Unity.

Philip Vickers
Director OCU

INTRODUCTION

Professor Ian Donald, CBE, MD, DSc, FRCS (Glas), FRCOG, Hon FACOG, pioneer of ultrasound diagnostics and author of *Practical Obstetric Problems*, was Regius Professor of Midwifery at the University of Glasgow until 1975. He is Honorary Fellow of the American College of Obstetricians and Gynecologists, and has been awarded the Eardley Holland Gold Medal by the Royal College of Obstetricians and Gynaecologists, the Victor Bonney Prize by the Royal College of Surgeons of England and the Blair-Bell Gold Medal from the Royal Society of Medicine. The subject of his current research is the prediction of ovulation.

1

INTRODUCTION

(to Second Edition)

PROFESSOR IAN DONALD

The subject of in-vitro-fertilisation started simply enough as a means of circumventing incurably blocked Fallopian tubes in women faced with the tragedy of infertility. It was rewarded six years ago with the successful birth of Louise Brown.

Since that day, techniques of artificial reproduction in both humans and animals have multiplied in a number of directions, by no means all of them acceptable to society. Like atomic fission they are here to stay and it is feared that codes of ethical medical practice will not be able to control their use and abuse. This does not mean that we should not press for effective legislation which is of paramount importance.

Christians cannot deny or shrug off their responsibilities. Indeed society must make up its mind about how far it will go along with Aldous Huxley's prophetic *Brave New World*. In the meantime attitudes may become polarised before they are properly informed and already the subject has rapidly extended to such matters as certain types of male infertility, transmissible genetic defect and the intrusion of a third party into the marital relationship, either in the form of donated sperm or ova, and varieties of surrogate parenthood.

The problem of what to do with spare human embryos now surplus to the needs of childless couples already looms large and in the background to all this lie the experimental opportunities for altering the nature of man as well as of animals.

Test-Tube Babies — A Christian View was originally pub-

3

lished in May 1984, a few weeks ahead of the Warnock Committee's report to HM government. It was based on a series of papers presented at a meeting convened by the Order of Christian Unity at the Royal Society of Medicine on 23 May 1983.

Recent developments

Since that meeting, events have arisen at an ever-accelerating rate. In this time there has been a modest improvement in the success rate of in-vitro-fertilisation restricted to certain types of infertility, which is welcome. To some extent this has been achieved by the fertilisation of up to three female ova for simultaneous placement in the mother's uterus. The use of pituitary stimulating hormones has enabled multiple ova to be retrieved, instead of just one, and the process of retrieval has been greatly facilitated by the use of an aspirating needle under ultrasonic echo guidance, thus obviating the need for laparoscopy under general anaesthesia. This favours selection of ova and, hopefully, makes multiple fertilisations of whole batches superfluous. The recent examples of four and six babies being delivered by one woman resulted from large numbers of fertilised eggs, with consequences highly undesirable both medically and socially.

So far so good but, not withstanding all this, the failure and disappointment rate remains high at around three quarters in even the most experienced units and there is little comfort for the majority, now worse off in hope as well as pocket.

Less welcome to most are present attempts to set up commercial surrogate agencies, charging, it is said, up to £24,000, to secure the hiring of another woman's womb to carry and then part with the child to the infertile woman, if possible inseminated by her husband. This is already profitable business in the USA and in this country there is no law to prevent it.

Freezing and storage of human embryos is already becoming commonplace and there is at present no limit to the duration of such cold storage. It is not difficult to imagine a sort of emporium, as is growing up in Australia, of hundreds of frozen human embryos with, presumably, catalogued genetic details awaiting claimants or customers, or failing that, experimentation to justify their very expensive upkeep. In the meantime a millionaire couple, who have had two embryos waiting to be collected in Melbourne, have been killed in an air crash and the question of inheritance has to be considered. It is even alleged

4

that they may result from donated sperm and there are already other children to consider from previous marriages.

The first freeze-thaw success was reported from Australia in March 1984 and more are known to be on the way. Furthermore a baby developed from an ovum donated by another woman has already been born there.

In England a human embryo has already been grown outside the womb for 13 days and there is a demand for six week old embryos as soon as research makes them available. Two surrogate mothers have already been hired and it remains to be seen what would happen if, having gone through the hazards of pregnancy and labour, their babies will be willingly given up. Any contract is likely to be unenforceable at law. A handicapped or deformed baby might be rejected by all concerned. Whose responsibility?

Embryo transfer by a flushing technique is now established in humans as has long been the case in the veterinary world. The first embryo transfer was achieved in rabbits in 1980. By 1920 it was already commonplace. Since then it has extended to breeding large numbers of genetically desirable lambs and calves born to common or garden surrogate mothers, and the profitable yield can be further increased by drug superovulation in the biological mothers.

Applied to humans this is a sophisticated form of surrogacy in reverse, in which the male partner of an infertile woman impregnates another woman and her very early five day old embryo is flushed out with the latest catheter technique from Sweden using the overfull urinary bladder to straighten out the genital canal. This entails no more than an outpatient attendance. The embryo's transfer to the infertile woman is then made at the same phase of the endometrial cycle to increase the chances of embedding. Interim freezing might help here. This is just a variant of the extra-corporeal IVF technique and has all the "merit" of technical adultery with no doubts as to the supposed paternity of the offspring. In the USA an attempt has been made to establish a lucrative business centre, complete with patent applications (which may well be refused); but 30,000 to 50,000 candidates a year are anticipated at 10,000 dollars per patient. Big business indeed and better than cattle breeding.

It is worth watching developments in the veterinary world because new techniques here are ultimately applicable to

5

humans. Indeed the plight of the infertile couple may be more of an excuse than a reason for much irrelevant research.

Experimentation

Clamour for this is bound to grow as scientific technology accelerates its momentum. Even the Warnock Committee was unable to agree about what degree of protection should be given to the human embryo. A majority upheld the view that experimentation was in order up to the fourteenth day of age. This is a fatuous inconsistency seeking to differentiate the rights of a 13 day embryo from those of a 15 day old one (as if any scientist would obey such a limit if he felt he was on the trail of something interesting). The supposed ability first to be able to feel pain is a sentimental, anatomical nonsense and is irrelevant, as is also the question of parental consent. It could as easily be applied to the anaesthetised and handicapped newborn and to the senile demented. This century has already witnessed this philosophy in Nazi Germany. In any case society can hardly be sentimental or squeamish about the 14 day old embryo when it tacitly accepts the evisceration and piecemeal extraction of fully formed babies at 24 weeks or more as a method of abortion under one and the same anaesthetic and euphemistically known in the USA as *D & E* (Dilatation and Extraction). This is offered by some as an alternative to induction of abortion to be followed by delivery itself of a designedly stillborn baby.

It is expensive to keep spare embryos deep-frozen indefinitely and, as an alternative to throwing them away a case is made out for making experimental use of them. Already in the UK 50 human embryos have been created and grown specifically for research, the ova being supplied by women being sterilised "for free" in return and the sperm from men undergoing vasectomy. After reaching the 2–4 cell stage they are dissected for chromosome analysis.

Even the ability of human sperm to fertilise hamster ova is now accepted up to the two cell stage as a test of male fertility.

Meanwhile veterinary technology races ahead. A sheep/goat hybrid has been bred in Cambridge and demonstrated on television a few months ago, with the boast that there were eight more like it. Likewise the delivery of a baby zebra from a donkey or horse was shown with the given reason that this was a way to prevent zebras as a species from dying out.

Most sinister of all new developments for the very immediate

6

future are the prospects for sex selection. It would hardly be an effective way of stamping out sex-linked disease since, by favouring the female progeny in a given union, it would merely be transferring the problem in the carrier state to the next generation. The Warnock Committee mentioned the possibility of a "do-it-yourself" sex selection kit and felt that the social problems which might ensue from its use should be "kept under review". With ever diminishing family sizes the inevitable preponderance of males, especially in the third world, would be disastrous.

Fertilisation in vitro is usually about 80 per cent successful. It is implantation which provides the technical difficulties at present. These are often blamed on chromosomal faults or numerical deficiencies. At present these can only be identified by cloning, i.e. removing one totipotential cell from the early embryo and culturing it to enable chromosome studies to be carried out, the remainder of the embryo being frozen until a verdict, one way or the other can be obtained from the cloned twin which is then discarded and the original embryo implanted or destroyed as thought appropriate.

If detailed genetic change could be found responsible for a given disease, an appropriate piece of DNA could be radioactively labelled to act as a gene probe applied to a detached cloned embryo. However, as yet, separating a two cell embryo has not been as safely achieved in the human as in animals. But it is still early days and the whole field of genetic engineering is only just beginning and "breeding according to specification" may not be so very far off.

Indeed with gene "therapy" and nuclear substitution the very nature of man could one day be altered and cloning could facilitate it on a grand scale.

It has been argued that both education and health care profoundly influence man's life already; true, but they do not alter man's individual identity.

Ectogenesis
An embryo, or foetus, does not need the inside of a uterus in which to develop provided it can be properly supplied with the necessary nutrients including oxygen and the riddance of its waste products. But at present there is a time gap between the latest day on which it can do without a placental circulation and sufficient development thereof to establish a circulatory by-pass

via the cannulated umbilical cord as is already being attempted. This time gap is likely to be progressively shortened with the advance of science. Meanwhile the use of a related surrogate mammal, such as a chimpanzee, may meet the requirement in order to mature an embryo which has been the subject of experimentation, since, outside institutions of a certain type, no ordinary woman would agree to carry the object of an experiment through to term. In the case of animals the question of "informed consent" does not arise.

Spare part surgery
The idea of cultivating the human foetus at some future date to meet a consumer demand for spare part surgery is horrifyingly callous, yet such has been suggested, however remote the prospect might at present seem.

Warnock Report inadequacies
This is a thoughtful document, beautifully written but weak in many of its sixty-three recommendations and frankly atheistic and amoral in some. It invokes the setting up of a Statutory Licensing Authority to apply controls which are clearly recognised as necessary. In fact it would allow embryos under controlled conditions to be kept alive, observed, frozen, stored (up to a maximum of ten years) and experimented upon up to 14 days and animal/human hybridisation limited to early stages.

Such a licensing authority, to be at all effective, would require a whole army of inspectors, each as knowledgeable as the members of the teams being inspected, which is most unlikely, and at an epoch when attempts to reduce rather than expand the bureaucracy it would be impossible to supervise more than a very few units. Collusion and confusion of the public would be inevitable. To do the Committee justice, its terms of reference were thought not to include the subject of abortion.

Artificial Insemination from Donor (AID) is recognised as having grown up in society in an entirely uncontrolled sort of way (which should warn us enough of how easily we can be presented with the fait accompli) but the Report is particularly concerned with the falsity which results in the birth certificate details of the offspring. The term "By Donation" is recommended where the "parent" of the child is not part of his originating source. This may be helpful in tracking genetic disease but must appear very disturbing to the youngster finding it on his birth certificate.

Attitude of the public
Thanks to the coverage by the media the interest and awareness of the public in such an intimate subject as human reproduction has been probably better informed than it is on such subjects as disarmament and even coal mining. The Order of Christian Unity therefore commissioned a nationwide MORI Poll* and many of us were surprised at how few, relatively, came under the "don't know" columns. The results presented here in graphic form have convinced us that we are not alone in our concern about some future developments and of the need to exercise some control over scientific technology's Gadarene descent.

IN-VITRO FERTILISATION

Q Do you think doctors and scientists should or should not be allowed to . . .
Fertilise a woman's ova outside her body in order to put the two to four-day old embryo produced back in her body?

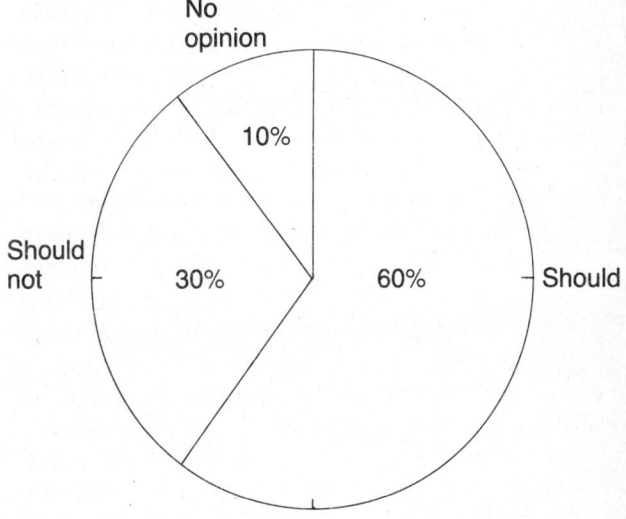

Technical note on MORI
MORI interviewed a representative quota sample of 1878 respondents aged 18 plus in 175 sampling points throughout Great Britain. All interviews were conducted face to face 19–23 July 1984 and data were weighted to the known demographic profile of the population.

SURROGATE MOTHERHOOD

Q Do you think doctors and scientists should or should not be allowed to . . .

Put one woman's two to four-day old embryo into the womb of another woman so she can carry the child for the original mother?

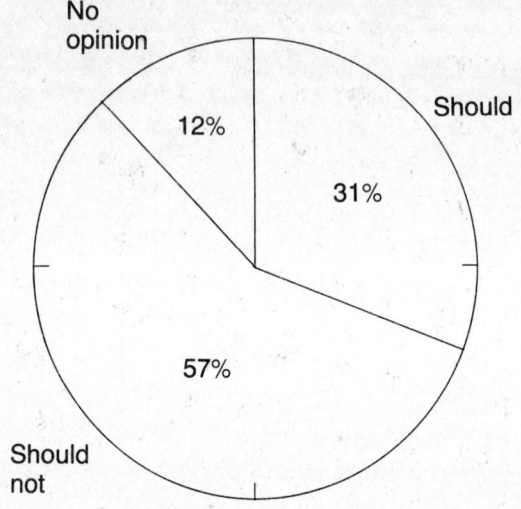

SCIENTIFIC RESEARCH

Q Do you think doctors and scientists should or should not be allowed to . . .

Fertilise human ova outside the mother's body for the sole purpose of creating human embryos for scientific and medical research?

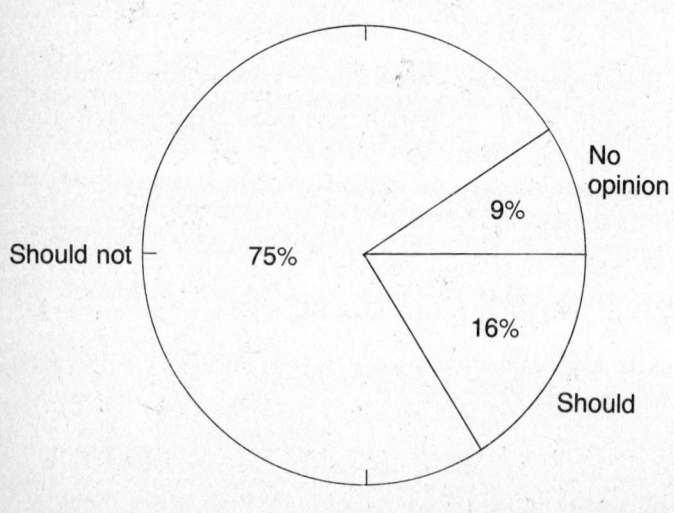

INTER-SPECIES BREEDING EXPERIMENTS

Q Do you think that experiments which involve the fertilisation of animal ova with human sperm, or human ova with animal sperm, to create a cross-bred embryo, should be allowed, or should such experiments be banned by law?

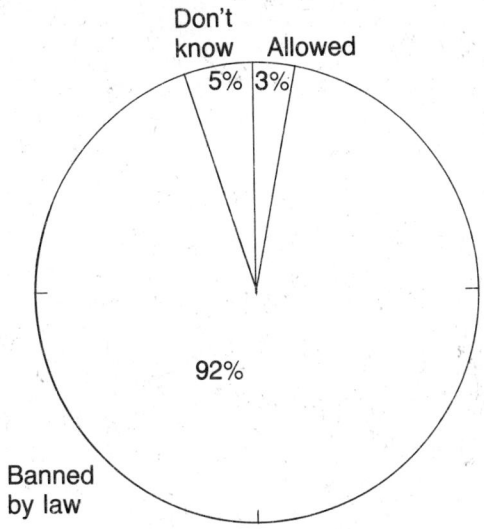

An Australian expert is reported as saying that test-tube babies are better than normally conceived children. This could militate against the welcome due to a naturally conceived child. It is bold talk since there has been no time yet in which to evaluate any long term effects on such children, physical or psychological, but the call from such authorities to educate the public to accept artificial methods of reproduction is a good example of brain washing. There is, however, no danger of the human race dying out from infertility!

Christian attitude
Some reviews of the first edition have criticised us for not dealing clearly with what the Christian attitude should be towards many of the spin-off abuses to which IVF lends itself. Now it must be quite clear that Christians everywhere would be guided by what Christ Himself would have done had He been a 20th century scientific technologist and not a carpenter.

Bearing in mind the purposes for which marriage was ordained, and about which He was uncompromisingly clear,

11

we recognise that He would not have accepted, for example, third party intrusion into the marital relationship, nor the parenthood of lesbians or homosexuals. The creation of man in His Father's image would not have accepted bio-engineering techniques inflicted on even the least of His children. He devoted much of His life to curing infirmity, including that which had afflicted its victims from their birth up. He did not destroy them nor deny their very existence. Instead His insistence on Faith was absolute, even to moving mountains — Faith in God's interest and loving care.

Outside our own faith, however, some sort of control is clearly necessary where none at present exists. In particular human rights, especially those of the baby, must be protected.

The issues are so complex that the Order of Christian Unity earnestly seeks a halt to experimentation on human life until the public as a whole, and Parliament in particular, do not find themselves on a slippery slope which they can no longer hope to remount.

IAN DONALD

31 October 1984
Paglesham, Essex

TECHNICAL HISTORY
OF IVF

Professor James Scott, MD, FRCS, FRCOG, is head of the Department of Gynaecology, University of Leeds. From 1977 to 1980 he was Chairman of the Scientific Advisory and Pathology Committee of the Royal College of Obstetricians and Gynaecologists. He is in the forefront of research into the immunology of pregnancy.

2

TECHNICAL HISTORY OF IVF

PROFESSOR JAMES SCOTT

In this paper it is my intention to try to put the major steps of in vitro fertilisation into perspective in relation to other scientific developments which have occurred in recent years in relation to human conception and embryonic development and the whole field of infertility. I will endeavour, as far as possible, not to stray into the realms of conjecture.

I should make my own position clear from the outset. I functioned myself, a matter of a decade or so ago, as a mere technician collecting ova for in vitro fertilisation. I therefore have no, or had no, basic fundamental objection to the procedure. Since then I have not been involved in any specific way. I have, however, seen the picture developing and have gradually become aware of the fundamental ethical problems that may arise as a consequence of it.

Matters have to be seen in relation to the whole problem of infertility. One of the noblest of human desires is to have a family. It is therefore one of the saddest situations the doctor has to face when he has a couple who desperately want to have their own children and find this impossible. Over the past twenty or thirty years there have been a series of major advances in this field. In vitro fertilisation is the most publicised and the most exciting of them, but many others have been of great importance.

The basic principles of the technique can be understood by a

15

child doing school biology. An egg is taken from the mother's ovary which lies within her abdominal cavity and is placed in a laboratory container in ideal chemical and physical circumstances. Arrangements are then made to introduce a sperm, or team of sperms, and fertilisation is allowed to take place. Once fertilised and the ovum has started dividing it is then transferred to the mother's womb. Although there are a lot of peripheral matters which must be considered, the basic technique is extremely simple.

It is important to realise that it is not a technique to overcome all forms of infertility but is merely appropriate for the small proportion of cases where there is absence of, or irreparable damage to, the fallopian tubes. There may be a few supplementary indications but not many.

When considering infertility, its investigation and treatment, it is only in terms of a couple that the term makes any sense. In investigating infertility we investigate the production and transport of the one gamete to where it can meet the other. The gamete is a term which covers both sperm and ovum, the male seed and the female egg. It is relatively easy to determine the production and conduction of the male gamete. It is merely a question of taking a little seminal fluid, possibly after intercourse, and seeing that the sperms are reaching their destination; in the female it can be much more difficult. When it comes to treatment on the other hand, failure of gamete production in the female can often be very easily corrected by giving gonadotrophins. (Gonadotrophins are the hormones produced by the endocrine part of the brain, the pituitary, which stimulate production of the eggs or sperm.) Treatment of failure of male gamete production, on the other hand, is extremely difficult.

Another aspect that should be borne in mind when considering this problem is the 'spin off' that there has been from research related to in vitro fertilisation upon other aspects of fertility problems. A great deal has been discovered about the production of gametes, about their transport and about the ideal conditions for the occurrence of fertilisation.

Similarity to space exploration

Creating man in the laboratory has got a similar sort of fascination to putting man on the moon and it is interesting to note that in the field of space research the effort of putting man on the moon has had a similar 'spin off' into the development of aeronautics. In many ways fertilisation is a remarkably similar sort of process to space exploration. For fertilisation, the human ovary shoots off its egg into what for it is virtual outer space, in this case the peritoneal cavity. The male gamete is introduced to the vagina at intercourse and by some quite miraculous processes that we do not really understand even to-day, makes its way towards the peritoneal cavity. There, or in the fallopian tube, sperm and ovum come together eventually. These two 'space-craft', first functioning independently, ultimately unite and undergo a 'soft landing' in the uterine cavity.

Various technical matters have contributed to the process. I have mentioned stimulation of the ovaries with drugs such as gonadotrophins when there is a failure of normal production. Gonadotrophins (or a synthetic drug clomiphene) are also used with in vitro fertilisation, even when there is no failure of ovulation, to produce 'super-ovulation'. By deliberately producing or inducing excessive production of gonadotrophins it is possible to ripen a multiplicity of ova simultaneously. This is useful for the technical aspects of recovering eggs for in vitro fertilisation. If there is only one ovum it may not be accessible but if there is a bunch of them, nearly always one or several will be accessible. There are also advantages on the laboratory side of having several ova to work with at the time of fertilisation and if the fertilisation (or fertilisations) should be successful then there will be a number of fertilised ova (early embryos) to replace. That of course immediately moves us into a new and major area of problem which I shall consider later.

Peritoneoscopy, or laparoscopy, is the passing of an instrument into the peritoneal cavity to look at the ovaries to see the development of the follicles. This was the basic line of interest which Steptoe originally had in the sixties. He then moved on to apply this facility in relation to collecting ova for fertilisation as the technique may be combined with passing a fine aspirating needle into the follicle(s) in the ovary and withdrawing the ova at the appropriate time.

Other developments include better techniques for assessing the timing of ovulation. Here Professor Donald's work in the field of ultrasonics has had its applications, alongside highly sophisticated chemical methods of assessing ovulation.

The chain of events all stems from the union of the ovum and the sperm which we call technically 'syngamy' (i.e. the coming together of the two gametes). There is then a conceptus which

17

goes on to be an embryo, a fetus, then a child and ultimately an adult. These are all stages of progressive development without rigid divisions. A lot of scientific work has gone into the development of the ideal physical and chemical laboratory environment for the occurrence of fertilisation and the early development of the conceptus. Assuming that this has occurred and that the fertilised ovum has started dividing there is then the question of re-implantation or implantation. People often talk loosely about 're-implantation' and 'donation'. The ovum has, of course, never been implanted before so there is strictly no question of re-implantation. It is an ovum which has been collected before fertilisation which is being re-implanted only in the sense that, in the great majority of cases, it is going back into the womb of the woman from whom it derived. The term 'ovum donation' generally refers to an ovum from another individual which is implanted in another woman's womb after fertilisation — whether 'mother' is the correct word here one can debate. This is, in a sense, the very earliest possible form of adoption.

Artificial insemination

Artificial insemination with the husband's sperm (A.I.H.) is a relatively easy procedure. It has long been practised and has long been widely accepted ethically. It may be thought of as the male equivalent of ovum collection and re-implantation in the female. It just so happens that with the female the techniques and the technology are vastly more complicated.

Donor insemination (A.I.D.) has gone on for a considerable time. Some 18,000 patients were started on donor insemination in the United Kingdom last year. Here sperm other than those of the husband are used for the donation. Ethically it is of course a different problem and it is one broadly corresponding to ovum donation. Donor gametes may be used to overcome a genetic problem or where one parent cannot produce them. Certainly there has been a broad acceptance of male gamete donation and it could be argued that there is therefore no argument against donation of ova, a fertilised ovum or an embryo.

One of the greatest problems that has come forward as in vitro fertilisation programmes have gone on, has been that arising from the creation of multiple embryos as a consequence of the hyper-stimulation techniques referred to previously, which improve tremendously the success rate of the whole procedure. It is possible to implant more than one to produce

18

twins or perhaps even triplets. Any order of multiple pregnancy beyond that level, however, is regarded as unreasonable particularly as it severely reduces the prospect of the mother carrying the implanted embryos to full term and having live babies - quite apart from the problems of managing the whole brood should they survive.

Frozen embryos

So the difficult question is what should be done with these 'spare' embryos (or, put another way, spare human beings)? If fertilisation has occurred successfully, is it not perfectly reasonable that the unneeded embryos should be kept? If deep frozen appropriately, they can be used in a subsequent cycle if the first implantation has not been successful or if the pregnancy miscarries at an early stage. These later attempts at implantation may be made without having to subject the mother to the risks and stresses of further peritoneoscopy to collect other ova. This view may seem reasonable but only superficially; there are many problems to be reckoned with.

The issue of freezing is therefore a major one. In our own practice we have been involved from time-to-time in collecting sperm from unfortunate married men who have not yet had a family but are afflicted by tumours which necessitate either radical surgery or radical radiation which, in either case, inactivates the testicles and produces sterility. If sperm is collected before this is done, it can be stored and can thereafter be used to father his own children. On the face of it this seems a perfectly reasonable procedure to most people. But as one progresses to other circumstances and other techniques there are obviously inherent, major and difficult problems with freeze-storing of gametes or embryos.

Not only is nature adapting and developing continuously, but our basic knowledge of the fundamental facts of nature and of reproduction, particularly fertilisation, are increasing day-by-day. Some quite extraordinary developments have taken place in the past decade or two in this area that it is only right we should have these in mind when we are discussing these subjects. Of particular importance is the technique of cloning. Once the fertilised ovum has divided you can take the cells, separate them, and from these grow two individuals, or more than two. Nature can, in fact, do a form of reverse cloning. From double fertilisation it can produce a single embryo.

19

Equally if there are two acts of syngamy it is possible for there to be dual paternity of a single individual, which is a startling idea to the lay person. I am not aware that it has been proved for singleton human pregnancies but it has been proved quite recently in a twin pregnancy that two fathers were involved. How nature manages to organise 'reverse cloning', two sets of cells coming together and forming an individual, is quite beyond understanding. Such individuals have been identified because they have got cells with 'XX' and 'XY' chromosome complements. In other words, as XX is the female complement and XY is the male complement they are chromosomally neuter. This may confuse a little but it does get across a message which may be important that Nature herself does not have many absolutely rigid rules.

Nature has also come up with what may be called reverse immaculate conception in relation to one of the most extraordinary forms of pregnancy that we have, hydatidiform mole. If one were to ask a biologist what he would regard as being the chromosomal complement of an immaculate conception he would I think say it was an individual who had two complements of chromosomes both derived from the mother. These hydatidiform mole pregnancies, however, have got quite the reverse, *a double contribution of chromosomes from the father but none whatever from the mother*. Yet the mother acts as host to this bizarre conception.

Another matter relevant to the problem on which a lot of new information has recently become available is that of high early conception loss. It has provoked a lot of discussion and has worried a lot of people. There are many figures around which range from a few per cent to 70 or 80 per cent for the number of early conceptions that abort. The latest figure from Newcastle is a little less sensational than some of the earlier ones. When special, sophisticated tests for the early occurrence of pregnancy are used it appears that about eight per cent abort never having been recognised clinically as pregnancies.

Whether these actually undergo implantation or not is another matter about which there is very little information. It is assumed that they undergo implantation although there is no positive proof of this. It does not seem to me to be a very fundamental issue although it clearly worries a lot of people who use it as an argument to indicate that early embryos are very much disposable. I feel that it is only an extension of what

20

paediatricians have known for a long time that the very early phases of extra-uterine life are dangerous; if this is projected backwards, the early stages of intra-uterine life close to the time of conception are *very highly dangerous*. This is related to something very badly taught in medical schools, namely the simple fact that human life is uniformly fatal! (There is a nice story about the paediatrician who was very keen on emphasising this tremendous hazard of early life and who was asked to give a talk on the subject somewhere in Scotland. He worked up to his great climax, which was that 'The first hour of life is the most dangerous!' at which point there was a voice from the back of the hall, from a grey-haired wizened old man, who said, 'Aye laddie, but the last hour's pretty dodgy too!')

Womb leasing

Surrogate motherhood or 'womb leasing' is another very emotive area, not necessarily related specifically to in vitro fertilisation. It has been employed in different ways and to mean different things. It can mean implanting an ovum into a mother's womb when she cannot provide her own ovum or the reverse, putting an ovum into a particular woman's uterus from another woman who has not, for example, a uterus which can carry it. This could be regarded as the equivalent, only at a different stage of development, of the wet nurse so well-known in history.

Finally, there is the question of research on artificially produced human embryos. Where do we stand with that? Research obviously has gone on with in vitro fertilised ova. The question is, how and where one draws the line. Sperms are easily available and have been used in research for decades. Why not ova, now available, and why not both together as the fertilised ovum? These are the sort of matters to which we have to turn our attention today.

FUTURE POSSIBLE USES AND ABUSES OF IVF

Dr David White. An Immunologist, Dr White is Senior Research Fellow at the Department of Surgery, University of Cambridge. He was responsible for the development of Cyclosporin A, the drug which has revolutionised the treatment of Leukemia and greatly increased the success of transplant surgery.

3

FUTURE POSSIBLE USES AND ABUSES OF IVF

DR DAVID WHITE

When I was invited to present a short talk at the Royal Society of Medicine on the possible future uses and abuses of in vitro fertilisation I looked forward to the project with some enthusiasm. A scientific presentation is rigorously bounded by the data and its interpretation. Here I was being asked to look into the future where no data yet exists and since one individual's speculations on that topic are as valid as any others I felt safe from criticism. In retrospect this was a naive view for several reasons. Firstly, I wrongly assumed a degree of understanding and acceptance of the scientific principles involved which in fact did not exist. To discover that there were gynaecologists who did not know what an allophene was came as something as a surprise. Secondly, I found that moral values were placed on scientific procedures usually because of unfortunate associations with the terminology used to describe them. For example, cloning is a routine biological procedure used in many laboratories for preparing homogeneous populations. Yet, for undefined reasons, the term and by extension the procedure, have taken on sinister implications.

Finally, despite substantial caveats during the presentation, many accepted predictions as fact. In particular, I discussed the possibility of creating new species and, as an example, I chose the possibility of creating a new underwater species with human characteristics. Trying to imagine possible new species that the genetic engineer might be able to create is somewhat like contemplating infinity. My choice of example was not guided by a desire to sensationalise or trivialise though in the event this turned out to be the end result. This choice was based on the principle that amphibians are particularly amenable to genetic engineering procedures and it is possible to produce their products in large numbers.

The manuscript which follows is essentially an annotated version of the recording of the talk I gave at the Conference. In editing it I was tempted to censor all reference to the possibility of creating new species since this example quoted out of context has caused me much embarrassment. However, I believe the possibility of creating new species really will come about in the next 30 years, and so I feel obliged to leave this section of the talk uncensored. Whether my choice of example is foolish or not only time will tell.

The ethics of creating mutant species containing human genetic information I am unqualified to comment on. In the final analysis everyone has to decide for themselves what they regard as acceptable to their own consciences and to the collective consciousness of a civilised society. I hope that the following report will assist them in this decision by giving a glimpse of what I think the future might hold.

Future possible uses and abuses of IVF and the manipulation of the human genome

Almost exactly 30 years ago two Cambridge post-graduate workers, Watson and Crick, published their now famous seminal paper on the structure of deoxyribonucleic acid [1]. In all it is only 880 words long. However, it has probably changed the science of biology and the potential of medicine more fundamentally than any other single observation. Watson and Crick wrote in their opening paragraph

"We wish to suggest a structure for the salt of deoxyribonucleic acid. This structure has novel features which are of considerable biological interest."

With this understatement they predicted the future growth and development of molecular biology to its present status. In this presentation I have tried to predict where this science might lead over the next thirty years, particularly in relationship to the use of in vitro fertilisation and the possibilities that arise from

26

this for the potential to manipulate the genes within the fertile ovum. Since it is impossible for me or anyone else to predict the future, the context of this talk is, by definition, speculative. Because of my brief to look at the future this talk also has little to do directly with in vitro fertilisation since that, as they say, is now history. For example, the potential for surrogate motherhood or womb renting already exists. So also exists the methodology for cloning or the production of multiple identities. I shall term these multiple genetic identities "true cloning". The principle involved is that a fertilised ovum is grown in culture. The cells formed are then separated into individual cells. With further culture these then grow so that each one will form a new individual, idential genetically to all the others derived from that initial fertilisation. This process can, in theory, be repeated several times so that one can produce large numbers of genetically identical individuals. The future potential from the development of this methodology is clear. You could have quads or quins perhaps all with different mothers but all having the same genetic identity. If this technology were to be combined with liquid nitrogen storage then clones could vary in their biological age. Indeed the frivolous notion that a woman could give birth to her twin sister may be contemplated.

Another possibility that stems from this ability to separate cells from the fertile ovum is that they can be used to identify the sex or indeed any other genetic trait or disease which will be present in the rest of the clone. Thus, clones with genetic defects can be identified and discarded.

Sex selection post fertilisation is thus a possibility. Another possibility that may be achieved is sex selection prior to fertilisation either in vivo or (less practically) in vitro. It may be that in the future techniques will be developed which will select out the sperm determining one particular sex and then allow fertilisation to take place only from the selected population. Such a technique could clearly be of great benefit to agriculture. Its benefit to mankind is more difficult to judge and in many cultures might lead to a substantial imbalance of the sex ratio.

Looking further into the future one must consider the possible ways in which the genetic content of the fertilised ovum might be manipulated. Production of allophenes or tetraparentals is one such way this might be achieved. The production of such hybrids is a routine laboratory procedure for those working with rodents.[2] Without describing the details of the technique, the priniciple it involves is the mixing together of the cells from the fertile ova of several sets of individuals, usually two sets of parents. Hence the term tetraparental or four parents. There is however no absolute restriction on the use of four individuals although to use more is uncommon. The cells that are mixed together then re-establish themselves randomly as a single blastomere giving an offspring which is an unequal mix of the two F1 types. It is unclear what innate restrictions there are on producing cross species allophenes. Indeed when one considers the genetic parentage of the mule one wonders if there are any such barriers to cross species production. Thus one must speculate on the possibility of producing allophenes between species, a man/monkey cross for example. Reaggregation and fertility would undoubtedly be a problem but the concept should not be entirely dismissed out of hand.

In addition to the production of hybrids, there are a number of other technologies available for the insertion of extraneous genetic material into the mammalian genome. These do not rightly fall within the scope of this talk since they already exist and my brief is to look to the future. However a brief reference to these technologies might serve to assist the reader in coming to terms with the speculations that follow since for those not familiar with the developments in molecular biology, they might otherwise consider them unreasonable flights of fancy.

The acquisition of relevant genetic material for implantation is not an insurmountable problem; enzymes can be used which locate and isolate the relevant section of nucleic acid and once obtained, a gene can be persuaded to replicate itself in vitro. Indeed once the amino acid sequence of the expressed genetic product is known one can synthesise one's own genes to produce it. Nowadays there are even machines which will synthesise genes for you automatically.

The reimplantation of this genetic material into the mammalian gamete or embryo does not present insurmountable problems either. This may be done either by attaching the genes to a virus which will then infect the cell or by microinjection. The latter technique is currently the most popular procedure used for introducing genes into mammalian embryonic cells. The real difficulty that arises with attempts to create these transgenic mutants is that very often, the artificially inserted gene is either not incorporated into the genome of a sufficiently large enough percentage of the cells of the individual or is not

28

expressed as a characteristic. Some progress has already been made however in this field as the creation of a supermouse by Palmiter and his colleagues[3] has shown. More spectacular and technically more elegant was the production by Illmense and Hoppe[4] of mammalian clones. These workers essentially performed two different types of manipulation. In the first they removed the paternal genetic material from the embryo and replaced it with a replica of the maternal genes thus producing a new individual homozygous for half of the maternal genotype. In their second experiment the embryonic genome was completely removed and replaced with genes taken from a cell line of another mouse, thereby for the first time cloning the mammalian genome. So controversial were these experiments that they had to be validated by an external investigation.

I have already referred to cloning as an extension of twinning. It seems likely that it will in future be possible to use the techniques pioneered by Illmense to clone at the genetic level rather than the cellular level. This then gives rise to the possibility that clones could be derived from genetic information contained within the adult. Whether anyone should want to perform such a manipulation in man is a debateable matter. Leaving aside the fictional notions of armies of clones or millionaires perpetuating their own images, there are a few reasons why one should seek to provide such cloning techniques in man. Perhaps the procedure might prove more acceptable than artificial insemination by donor in cases of sterility which are due to inability to provide a functional gamete. It would seem likely however that such cloning techniques will in future be used to preserve genetic excellence produced by selective (and expensive) inter-breeding programmes. For example, in racehorses, where the inevitable high failure rate associated with such techniques might be more acceptable.

Another possible development that one must contemplate is the use of gene therapy. While the treatment of a patient by genomic manipulation falls outside the scope of this presentation, Williamson[5] in his excellent review of this subject, points out that such treatments might well have a better chance of success if the genetic rearrangement was performed on embryos after in vitro fertilisation and prior to reimplantation. Thus the elimination of such gene defects as cystic fibrosis might one day become a reality.

In this discussion of the manipulation of the human genome

it is important to stress that the species source of the novel genetic material is unimportant and that once incorporated into the genome this material will be inherited. Thus it is reasonable to speculate that by combining the techniques of genetic engineering and allophene production it should be possible to speed up the evolutionary process or steer it in new directions or even bypass it altogether and create either novel mutants or entirely new species. For example, the suggestion that it might be possible to colonise the sea by creating a hybrid amphibian mutant species containing human characteristics is just one of many possible scenarios that one could speculate about ad infinitum. Another possibility might be the production of a breed of animals expressing only human transplantation antigens on their cell surface, thereby providing a suitable source of organs for transplantation.

Finally I would like to consider the possibility of producing biologically active substances from specialised cell culture of embryonic material. It is possible that in the future one will be able to culture an embryo in certain conditions so as to produce cell lines grown from that embryo which will either possess biologically important properties or secrete biologically active products. Examples such as growth hormone or the islets of Langerhans come to mind immediately. Genetic engineers would argue that in most cases these embryonically developed lines could be discarded once they have yielded the necessary gene sequence and indeed this may well be the case.

I have tried to look forward over a time span of 30 years and speculate just what developments might take place. History teaches us that any such action is doomed to failure and nothing is more certain than that many of the predictions I have made here will never become technically possible. It is equally certain that many which I have not made will assume great biological importance or become regarded as commonplace.

I have tried to present these speculations without making any moral judgements. I have done so for several reasons; firstly, such judgements are at least in part a reflection of the times in which one lives, thus to impose today's standards on events which may occur in the future is a somewhat futile exercise. Secondly, I believe everyone should be allowed to apply their own informed moral judgements on such issues. Lastly, the techniques which must be developed for the speculations I have made here to become reality do not in themselves require moral judgement. It is the use to which they are put that requires careful scrutiny.

It has been suggested that embargos should be placed on certain areas of research because the technologies that they might develop would be open to abuse. I believe that to attempt to regulate the potential abuses that society might make of future scientific advances by prohibiting scientific enquiry would be to impose the wrong kind of restrictions on the wrong population of individuals for the wrong reasons. It is inevitable that where there are new frontiers to be crossed and new continents to be explored man will always wish to travel to these Brave New Worlds.

REFERENCES
1 Watson J. D. and Crick F. H. C. Nature *171* 737 (1953).
2 Minz B. Science *138* 594 (1962).
3 Palmiter et al. Nature *300* 611 (1982).
4 Illmense and Hoppe. Cell *23* 9 (1981).
5 Williamson R. Nature *298* 416 (1982).
6 Kobel H. R. and Du Pasquier. Developmental Immunobiology. Elsevier Amsterdam p 299 (1977).

GENETIC ENGINEERING:
TEST TUBE BABIES ARE BABIES

Professor Jerome Lejeune, MD, PhD, French geneticist, is Professor of Fundamental Genetics at the Faculty of Medicine, University of Paris. He is a member of the American Academy of Arts and Sciences and an Officier Ordre Nationale du Merit. He has also been awarded the Kennedy Prize. His publications include *Discovery of the Extra Chromosome in Trisomy 21* (mongolism), and research papers on human chromosomes and mental deficiency.

4
GENETIC ENGINEERING: TEST TUBE BABIES ARE BABIES

PROFESSOR JEROME LEJEUNE

The fundamentals of life

Life has a very, very long history but each individual has a very neat beginning, the moment of its conception. As it has been amply demonstrated, the whole biology of vertebrates teaches us that ancestors are united to their progeny by a continuous material link, for it is from the fertilization of the female cell (the ovum) by the male cell (the spermatozoa) that a new member of the species will emerge.

The material link is the thread-like molecule of DNA. This ribbon, roughly one meter long, is cut into pieces (23 in man), and each segment is carefully coiled and packaged in the form of a little rod, clearly visible under the microscrope, the chromosome.

As soon as the 23 maternal chromosomes encounter the 23 paternal chromosomes, the full genetic information, necessary and sufficient to spellout all the inborn qualities of the new individual is gathered.

Just as the introduction of a minicassette into a tape recorder will allow the reproduction of a symphony so the information included in the 46 chromosomes (the minicassettes of the life music) will be deciphered by the machinery of the cytoplasm of the fertilized egg (the tape recorder), and the new being begins to express himself as soon as he has been conceived.

The fact that the baby will develop himself for another nine months inside the womb is irrelevant to this point as in vitro fertlization has amply demonstrated.

The technicalities of fecundation

In natural conditions, the ripe ovum is expelled from the ovary by rupture of the follicle and is recovered by the fallopian tube. Inside this tube it migrates toward the uterus and en route encounters the sperm which, among millions of others, will fertilize it.

At the end of the journey the fertilised egg, already dividing feverishly, and organizing itself in a miniscule embryo of one millimeter and a half of diameter, accommodates itself inside the uterine mucosa (nidation); around six to seven days after fertilization has taken place. There, firmly implanting itself thanks to its chorionic villi, it will continue its growth until birth.

It is because normal fertilization occurs in a tube, with ovum and sperm floating freely inside the liquid, that test tube babies are possible. Indeed, in vitro fertilization uses a tube of glass instead of a tube of living tissue, but the process is, in other respects, identical.

Initially, artificial fertlization outside the maternal body has been proposed to circumvent some cases of feminine sterility. It happens that sometimes the fallopian tubes are blocked, most often as a sequela of a sexually transmissible disease. In such cases, the spermatozoa cannot reach the egg nor can the egg reach the uterus. To circumvent this block, the ripe egg is taken out by laparoscopy and put into a vessel containing appropriate medium. Addition of sperm will lead to fertilization.

The early embryo will be delicately transferred a few days later, through the cervix of the uterus so that it can pursue its development in the womb.

All of this explains why Dr Edwards and Dr Steptoe could witness, in vitro, the very beginning of the exceedingly young Louise Brown whom they replaced a few days later in the womb of her mother. Thanks to the fundamentals of life already known, they were totally assured that this little berry-looking being could not be a tumor nor an animal.

With the hundreds of cases already described in various countries of the world, a double evidence is now available, and for the first time, in our own species. The early human embryo is developing itself by its own virtue and it has an incredible viability[1].

Viability outside the womb

That the early human being is fully viable outside the maternal body is not a surprise but a confirmation of general principles.

Even in ordinary conditions, with a rather simple culture medium (the fluid of the fallopian tube), the early human embryo can pursue its own destiny for days, maybe a week, and manage its own organization. After one week implantation is a necessity but the viability of the early human being is such that even the uterine mucosa is not a prerequisite.

Up to two months implantation inside the fallopian tube is fully efficient. In these extra-uterine, ectopic pregnancies the tiny human being, smaller than the thumb, is perfectly developed. The only danger being that his continuous growth would rupture dramatically the walls of the tube which cannot extend as a uterus would. Even in the extreme case of extra-genital pregnancies, when the fetus anchors itself in the abdominal cavity directly on the peritoneum, the growth can be astonishingly normal for many months.

Protected by his life capsule, the zona pellucida first and later, the amniotic bag he constructs around himself, the early human being is just as viable and autonomous as an astronaut on the moon. Refuelling with vital fluids is required from the mother ship.

A purely artificial fluid supplier has not yet been invented. But if it were ever possible complete development outside the womb would ensue. Such "ectogenesis" would be the utmost proof that an embryo or a baby belongs to himself. If the bottle would argue that this baby is my property, no one would believe the bottle.

Time at a standstill

Careful refrigeration of living cells protecting their precious molecular edifice is of common use for long preservation. At a very low temperature, minus 190C in liquid nitrogen, the vibration of the atoms is quite restricted. Time is suspended so to speak.

Frozen sperm can thus be kept for years. If thawed carefully, they fully recover their fate as intrepid navigators. Banks of sperm are a common tool of industrial breeding.

The same is true for early embryos. Some mouse embryos, deep frozen and thawed, have managed after implantation to develop themselves into perfectly normal mice. No such experiment has yet been reported in our species. Proposals are numerous although their legitimacy is at least questionable.

Twins at will

If the zona pellucida is split and the embryo cleaved in two halves, each mass can be inserted in a separate zona pellucida.

Identical twins have thus been produced in cattle and in sheep. Some have proposed to do the same in man. Their rationale is not "a production line" but the possibility of checking the genetic make-up of one of the twins. The scenario goes as follows. One of the twins is deep frozen until further transfer at the proper time in a recipient uterus. The other twin is allowed to grow for a while and is then examined for its chromosomal constitution, normality of growth, and its various chemical properties. The spared twin will then be transferred if the sacrificed one is declared to be alright. If it is not the spared one will not be spared any longer. Supposedly, this procedure will give full insurance for successful childbearing even for a mother at risk due to chromosomal or genetic disease.

Simple arithmetic (see Annex) is not so optimistic. A success rate better than a few per cent can hardly be expected. As a mean, the egg donor should be tapped some twenty times for each successful pregnancy, an extremely heavy burden, not to speak of the 20 to 40 embryos who would not survive the whole experiment.

Wombs for hire

If properly kept in suspended life, there being no synchrony of ovarian cycles in the population, an early embryo could be transferred at any time in any recipient uterus. For example, a widow could accommodate a spared embryo fathered long ago by her departed partner. A candidate affected by an inheritable disease would welcome an egg from a healthy donor. A uterine foster mother could be hired if the true mother could not, for medical reasons, assume the pregnancy. Possibly a career woman could thus avoid the inconveniences of the pregnant state.

Surrogate pregnancy is a difficult issue. Should the foster mother be forced to give back the baby nine months later? Should she be deprived the right of voluntary termination of pregnancy if abortion is legal in her country? These questions are for lawyers. For the biologist no matter what the avowed pretext such practices would break the only assured link between generations. Up to now, in spite of all the uncertainties of passion, motherhood was an absolute certainty at delivery.

Sure enough the technique works in cattle. But, what is good for calves and cows may not be good enough for children and mothers.

Manipulated embryos

The full viability of the early being and its striving for life allow many experiments.

The cells of two different embryos can be mixed together. They thus cooperate in the making of a compound animal called a chimera. To the best of our actual knowledge, no compound mouse has yet been obtained from more than three cell lines mixed together[2]. During the first cleavages of the fertlized egg there is an odd stage of three primordial cells. Maybe this three-cells stage has something to do with the individualizing process.

It must be remembered that normally the zona pellucida prevents these admixtures. In a sense this bag protects our early private life. It is an open possibility that normally the human embryo hatches out of its zona pellucida only when its biological individuality is so strongly established that a chimeric accident is no longer to be feared.

But even if the mixing must be restricted to two or three cell lines, what about an 'artistic' embryo, an 'athletic' embryo, and a 'scientific' one fused together? Would not that create a kind of superman? Or, if DNA manipulation comes in what about embryos receiving special sequences, producing exceptional endowments?

These fictional experiments do not deserve discussion. These nursery tales for grown-ups can be rejected easily. To devise a man wiser than we are we should be already wiser than we can be!

As for the proposals of manipulating embryos in order to

recuperate spare parts for repairing children or adults, they are so farfetched that no critical analysis can be made. Conceivably, grafts of stem cells could be of theoretical interest. They are already taken from voluntary donors such as a bone marrow graft for example. In any event, specialized tissues are not yet detectable in pre-implantation embryos.

A sex of choice

As Brungs stated abruptly about the advent of generalized contraception and, later, of efficient in vitro fertilization, we have gone "from sex without babies to babies without sex." But, the sex of the baby still matters.

The choice of the king is a son for the first child and often for the second. The same is true for the layman, even for the suffragettes and now the feminists. All the opinion polls give the same answer: If free choice were given a formidable excess of males would result.

Fortunately no sieve is available to select preferentially the male sperms, carriers of the "Y" chromosome. Pre-sexing of the embryo is also quite out of sight.

If an acceptable technique was some day available the State could not remain indifferent in the face of such a foreseeable disaster as a woman-deprived population. Not to infringe upon free choice and not to favour anyone enormous computers would process the demands, producing optimal decisions. As demonstrated by Grouchy[3] the best equation is not too cumbersome to calculate. Toss a coin like before.

The very question

If our only goal is to help women who cannot procreate because of tubal difficulties, have we chosen the right track?

Let us return to technicalities. If, in reality, the early embryo is not an experimental material to be split, mixed, and manipulated, what is the interest of this trip of a few days in the outside world?

Dr Craft and his colleagues have already shown that the fertilized ovum can be implanted in the womb right away[4]. Could we not go even closer to physiological process? Possibly the egg could be placed in the uterus during laparoscopy with the sperm already being supplied by normal intercourse.

Why not study more closely the fluid of the fallopian tube? Would it not be the best medium for early development?

Research workers would be very wise to explore new avenues rather than automatically following the long detour of in vitro fertilization.

The future of medicine

Repeatedly, arguments have been put forward that in vitro fertilization would help cure a whole array of diseases including breast cancer. But all the available evidence points toward other directions of research as shown by three recent examples.

Among the genetic scourges afflicting humanity mental retardation is the most inhumane. It deprives patients of one of the most precious parts of our patrimony, the full power of thought.

Some ten per cent of the mentally retarded show a peculiar fragility of the "x" chromosome. Numerous examinations have shown that this fragility can be healed if the cells are cultivated in a medium containing various chemicals, a simple vitamin or folic acid and its derivatives are especially efficient[5]. If it is added to the regimen of the patients their chromosome gap seems to disappear as well. Moreover, preliminary clinical trials show that their mental status can be ameliorated partially[6].

The cure of the disease is not already at hand; but this is the first time that a chromosomal dissease and its deleterious consequences can be attacked without resorting to science fiction devices.

Another terrible disease resulting from imperfect closure to the neural tube in embryonic life seems also to be amenable to vitamin therapy. As demonstrated by Smithells[7] et al and confirmed by Laurence et al, vitaminotherapy, including folic acid, given in appropriate time to the mother at risk diminishes drastically the frequency of spina bifida. Here, again, no experiment on the embryo is required.

A third advance has been made on genetically transmitted anemias.

During in utero life, hemoglobin is produced by an array of different genes working one after the other:
the first during the embryonic stage,
the second in the fetus, and
the third in the whole adult life.
If this last gene is mutated, an abnormal hemoglobin is made (as in thalassemias or in sickle-cell anemia).

It happens that the silent genes can be 'woken up' by a special

41

chemical called azacytidine (Ley et al)[9] and take advantage of this property so that the patients, rather than suffering from their abnormal adult-type hemoglobin, start producing again their normal fetal type. This type of rejuvenation could be of great significance for therapy without any manipulation of embryos or the fetus.

Aldous Huxley, Wolfgang Goethe, and the newspaperman

A last question remains. Why is in vitro fertilization such a fascinating issue? Although the *Brave New World* is often quoted in this context, it is probably not the industrial production line of identical twins which is the key point. Aldous Huxley stressed another phenomenon. In that technological society, liberated from every taboo, the various dirty words were in current use. Nevertheless, the editors were obliged to reprint all the literature in order to remove the only incongruity which could not be pronounced, should not even be read, and was to be replaced by three points of suspension. This was the word 'mother'.

Motherhood a pure obscenity, an inversion of values, is a real danger Aldous Huxley has warned us about.

Another author, one of the greatest poets more than a century and a half ago, saw much further. With the 'Damnation of Dr. Faust' Goethe told of the tragic abandonment of the beloved, seduced and pregnant. In the second Faust the vision goes even deeper. After his pact with Mephistopheles Faust comes back to his old laboratory with his diabolic companion. They watch the successor of Faust producing an homunculus inside an alchemic vessel. The tiny creature escapes and floats in the air around the head of Dr. Faust who, guided as he is by this strange dream baby, has definitely lost his mind but not his imagination. After impossible love with the ghost of Helen of Troy Faust finally accomplishes his goal. He builds an empire, a fully technical society, with the magic help of Mephisto. At the very end he gives his last orders — to silence the little church bell, the only one still ringing in his whole empire, and to destroy the little cabin in which Philemon and Baucis are still the paragon of human love. When the silence comes, when Mephisto returns after having burned the old lovers in their cabin, then, sorrow invades the heart of the doctor.

Poets are beyond science. They see it from far away, but they feel much more than technicians could ever grasp. In such important matters it would possibly be very profitable for scientists and legislators to read the great authors once again.

Maybe, they could also rely on other writers who are much more accessible and living among us, the newspapermen. They too do not make science but see it from outside and their judgement is not taken lightly. They know that in vitro fertilization fascinates their readers. One journalist understood why. Trying to convey all the significance of what was going on he coined the term 'test-tube baby'. Sure enough, scientists objected — they had overlooked it — but the journalist knew better.

If any exploitation of the early human embryo is intrinsically repugnant, if everyone feels that those conducting experiments must absolutely respect these marvellously young human beings, it is for the scientific reason that a newsman discovered in an intuition of genius, test-tube babies *are* babies.

NOTES

[1]Lejeune, J. On the beginning of human life. Testimony before the Senate of the United States of America, Subcommittee on Separation of Powers, April, 13, 1981.

[2]Grouchy, J. de Jumeaux, Mosaiques, Chimeres et autres aleas de la fecondation humaine. MEDSI Edit. Paris 1980.

[3]Grouchy, J. de. Les nouveaux Pygmalions. Tauthier Villars Edit. Paris 1973.

[4]Craft, McLeod F., Green S., Djajanbalich, O., Vernard, A., Twigg, H. et Smith, W. 1982 - Birth following oocyte and sperm transfer to the uterus. Lancet ii, 1982, 773.

[5]Sutherland, G. R. 1979. Heritable fragile sites on human chromosomes 1. Factors affecting expression in lymphocyte culture. Am. J. Hum. Genet. 31. 125-135.

[6]Lejeune, J. Le metabolisme des monocarbons et le syndrome de l'X fragile. Bull. Acad. Nat. Med. 1981, 165.

[7]Smithells, R. W., Sheppard, S., Schorah, C. J., Selle, M. J., Nevin, N. C., Harris, R., Read, A. P., et Fieldink, D. W. Possible prevention of neural tube defects by periconceptional vitamin supplementation. Lancet i, 339-40, 1980.

[8]Laurence, K.M., James, N., Miller, N. H., Tennant, G. B. et Campbell, H. 1981. Double-blind randomized controlled trial on folate treatment before conception to prevent recurrence of neural-tube defects. Brit. Med.f J. 282, 1509-1511.

[9]Ley, T. J., Desimone, J., Anagnov, N. P., Keller, G. H., Humphries, B., Turner, P. M., Young, N. S., Heller, P., Nienhuis, A. W. 1982. 5-azacytidine selectively increases 8-globulin synthesis in a patient with B+thalassemia. New Engl. J. Medicine 307, 1475-1469.

Tentative estimation of the success rate of the whole process of implantation of a defrosted embryo after artificial twinning and genetic check-up of its sacrificed co-twin.

This process has five independent steps. The total likelihood is thus the product of the individual probabilities of success for each event.

(1) Successful recovery of the egg by laparoscopy and in vitro fertilization.

Let us take a 90 per cent chance of success, which seems a rather high standard.

(2) Splitting of the zona pellucida, splitting of the embryo, accommodation of each would-be twin in a new zona pellucida with good chances of survival of the two.

Let us take the very optimistic view that both twins do quite well in 50 per cent of the cases. (The records in animals are not that high by far.)

(3) Successful genetic check-up of the sacrificed twin after tissue culture and biochemical control.

Let us suppose 90 per cent are successes, a rate difficult to attain in examinations after amniocentesis in the second trimester of pregnancy.

(4) Successful freezing and thawing of the spared embryo.

No estimate can be given for it has not yet been reported in man. Let us take the optimistic view of 50 per cent. Such a success rate has never been reported in experimental animals, by far.

(5) Healthy development to full term of the spared embryo after its transfer in utero.

A value of 25 per cent can be assumed as a very favourable one, considering the available statistics published.

All together, the likelihood of the whole process is: $p = 0,90 \times 0,50 \times 0,90, 0,50 \times 0,25 = 0,05$.

Although this value of five percent is disputable, mainly because steps 2 and 4 are yet unknown, it can hardly be argued that it is a deliberate underestimate. Very likely, the chance of success of the full procedure would be quite a bit lower.

THE LEGAL IMPLICATIONS OF IVF

Mr Gerard Wright, QC, is noted for his achievement in getting index linked compensation for the victims of the Thalidomide tragedy.

5
THE LEGAL IMPLICATIONS OF IVF

MR GERARD WRIGHT, QC.

In discussing the legal implications of in vitro fertilisation I start from one basic proposition: that human life begins at conception. As a Christian lawyer my concern is to see what protection the law gives to human life when it is conceived in vitro. However before I embark on that specific topic I want to outline very briefly some of the legal problems which uncontrolled in vitro fertilisation may give rise to.

The simplest form of in vitro fertilisation is where an ovum is taken from a woman, fertilised with her husband's sperm in vitro, and then implanted in her womb. The mind boggles however at the possible permutations — I call them parental permutations — on that simple theme.

One permutation is where there is what is called sperm donation. Here the ovum is taken from the wife, but the sperm used to fertilise it is obtained from someone other than her husband. This practice can cause many legal problems. To list but a few, there is the problem of the resulting child's legitimacy and its right of inheritance. There may also be problems concerning maintenance of the child and custody and access, and these matters may involve the sperm donor as well as the reputed parents.

Another permutation arises when there is ovum donation. Here it is another woman's ovum that is fertilised with the husband's sperm and then implanted in his wife's womb. Thus, although she bears a child, she is not its biological mother. Here also knotty legal problems may arise of legitimacy, inheritance, custody and so on.

Whose baby is it?

Then there is what has been called womb leasing. Here the wife's own ovum and her husband's sperm are used but the resulting in vitro conceptus is then implanted in some other woman's womb. Whose baby is it when it is born? Must the biological parents accept it when it is born, even if it is born handicapped? Must the woman who bears the child hand it over to its biological parents? The scope here for human tragedy is immense, and legal solutions will have to be found for these appalling problems.

Even greater problems are about to be superimposed on those I have mentioned, for we now know that it is possible to deep-freeze an in vitro conceptus and then implant it. This poses such problems as the right of inheritance of a child born from an alien womb perhaps a generation after the death of its biological parents.

These are but *some* of the legal problems which in vitro fertilisation may give rise to. I do not intend to give the answers to any of them. The lawyers of the future may make their fortunes doing that. My object in outlining those problems is to give you some idea of the nature of the Pandora's Box which in vitro fertilisation will open if it is not carefully and strictly controlled.

The problems I have mentioned arise after the in vitro conceptus has been born from the womb in which it is implanted. What I want to consider with you now is the protection — if any — which the law gives to the living in vitro conceptus while it is unimplanted.

What we have to consider is not just the tiny blastocyst which at present lives for just a few days and dies if it is not implanted in a womb. We must also look to the future and assume that it will soon be possible to nourish the in vitro conceptus outside the womb, and that in time we will have a one month, a three month, conceptus in vitro. Indeed eventually perhaps there will be a fully mature baby that has never known a womb.

Protection of the law

What protection does the law give to the in vitro conceptus as it progresses, in vitro, from tiny blastocyst to fully developed baby?

Let us first consider Statute Law. There is no statute which gives any protection to the life of the in vitro conceptus at any stage of its existence in vitro.

The principal statutory provisions protecting the unborn are sections 58 and 59 of the Offences against the Person Act 1861. These provisions are directed against causing a woman to miscarry and, as no woman is 'carrying' the in vitro conceptus, these provisions do not protect it.

One might think that the Infant Life (Preservation) Act 1929 would protect the in vitro conceptus, at least in the later stages of its maturity. That Act however is concerned with 'causing a child to die before it has an existence independent of its mother'. As the in vitro conceptus is wholly independent of any mother, the Act does not protect it.

Finally the Abortion Act 1967 gives no help, for it concerns the termination of pregnancies, and here there is no pregnancy.

As no statute protects the life of the in vitro conceptus we must look to the Common Law for any protection there may be. In particular we must look at the law of murder which is a common law, not a statutory, offence.

May I stress that I am now entering upon uncharted territory, for the question of the life of the in vitro conceptus has not yet been considered by any Court. What I am about to do is to suggest, very tentatively, some ways in which the common law can be adapted to protect the life, the human life, of the in vitro conceptus.

The principle obstacle to protection is the traditional definition of murder. Way back in the Thirteenth Century that great jurist Henry Bracton said that it was murder to kill a child in the womb. Opinions changed however and by the time that Sir Edward Coke and others came to write treatises on the law in the Seventeenth Century it was agreed that the killing of a child in the womb was not murder. It was only murder if the child was fully born. Those writers therefore defined the potential victim of the crime of murder as 'a reasonable creature in esse' or 'in rerum natura'.

Now an in vitro conceptus is indeed 'in esse' or 'in rerum natura' because it is not in a womb. But is it what the law calls 'a reasonable creature'? I have sufficient faith in the common law of England, and in the Judges who mould and adapt it to changing circumstances, to predict with some confidence that once you have an in vitro conceptus which has plainly recognis-

49

able human shape and form and is plainly moving and alive, then the Courts will say: this is a reasonable creature and you commit murder if you destroy it. An in vitro conceptus will reach this stage by at least its third month of maturity. But before this stage destruction would not be murder.

But, if it is not murder to destroy the in vitro conceptus *before* it reaches this stage, is there no protection at common law for the life of the conceptus until it reaches this stage? I put forward very tentatively the view that there may be some protection.

In order to explain this view I must first deal with a statement made on 10 May 1983 by the Attorney General in the House of Commons. In making this statement the Attorney General was answering a question about the post coital pill. In summary he said that that pill was not illegal because it acted upon an *unimplanted* fertilised ovum. Logically one might think that if an unimplanted fertilised ovum carried by a woman in her body is unprotected by the law, it must follow that the unimplanted fertilised ovum which is in vitro is also unprotected by the law.

However I have two comments to make on the Attorney General's much publicised statement. The first is that his answer was specifically related to possible proceedings under the Offences against the Person Act 1861. He said that the word 'miscarriage' in that Act must be interpreted in accordance with the meaning which would have been given to it in 1861 when the Act was passed. This meaning he said did not include the expulsion from the womb of an unimplanted fertilised ovum. With all due respect to the Attorney General, he has been incorrectly informed as to the meaning attributed to the word 'miscarriage' in 1861. Reference to contemporary medical and medico-legal text books will demonstrate the Attorney General's error, for in 1861 the word miscarriage did include the expulsion of an unimplanted ovum. My first comment therefore is that the unimplanted fertilised ovum in a woman's body *is* protected by the Offences against the Person Act 1861, and the post coital pill is therefore illegal.

My second comment is that, even if the Attorney General's interpretation of the Offences against the Person Act 1861 were right, the matter does not end there. Abortion is not only an offence created by statute. Long before 1863, when the first statute against abortion was passed, there existed an offence at common law.

Common law

I have told you how in the Seventeenth Century Sir Edward Coke and others said that it is not murder to kill a child in the womb. Let me tell you more. What they said was that, whilst it was not murder, it was nevertheless 'a great misprision', that is to say a criminal offence at common law less serious than murder. This criminal offence at common law — you will find a precedent for an indictment in Chitty's Criminal Law — has never been abolished and it still exists.

Can this common law criminal offence be prayed in aid to protect the conceptus which, though living, does not yet have recognisable human shape or form? If one reads Coke and others it is apparent that the offence is committed if the child is 'quick'. But what does 'quick' mean? Most of you are familiar with the phrase 'the quick and the dead'. This gives the clue: quick means, quite simply, alive, living.

In the Seventeenth Century a fetus was thought to be alive, and therefore protected by the law, when its mother experienced the physical sensation known as 'quickening'. This sensation was accepted as evidence of life. I would suggest, however, that quickening is no more than an evidentiary test and that the underlying principle of the law — I hope to no one's surprise — is that human life is to be protected simply because it is human life.

What I suggest is that in the light of modern medical knowledge the law would in no way be subverted if we discarded the outdated and erroneous evidentiary test of quickening and said quite simply that it is a criminal offence at common law to destroy a conceptus because what you destroy is human life.

If what I suggest is acceptable, then the law protects the conceptus whether it is implanted or unimplanted, whether it is in the body of a woman or in vitro, and whatever its stage of maturity.

So far I have been considering whether the law protects the *life* of the in vitro conceptus. I want to look now at its general well-being to see if the law protects it from misuse. If one asks whether there is anything in law to prevent a scientist from doing what he likes — short of deliberate destruction — with the in vitro conceptus, I must answer with regret that there is nothing to control him.

Neither statute nor the common law forbids the fertilisation in vitro of a human ovum. Therefore the scientist may fertilise, with impunity, as many ova as he wishes. There is no law to compel him to implant any that he has fertilised. He thus has a choice. He may watch the conceptus die. That is not illegal. He may try to keep it alive for as long as possible for the benefit of his own researches. That also is not illegal. It follows that today we face the very real prospect of human life being deliberately brought into existence solely for the purpose of medical research, and there is no law to stop this from happening.

I would like to summarise briefly what I have been saying. The first point I have made is that uncontrolled in vitro fertilisation leads to quite appalling and, in human terms, tragic, legal problems once the conceptus is born. The second point I have made is that the law is far from clear as to whether the in vitro conceptus is protected from deliberate destruction. All that I have been able to do is to show how the law might — I put it no higher — be adapted to protect the life of the in vitro conceptus. Finally, I have made the point that there is no principle of law which prevents human life from being brought into existence at the whim of the scientist and for no other reason than to further his research.

Need for legislation

I am firmly of the view that in the situation I have been describing what is needed is not ethical guide lines drawn up by some committee of the B.M.A. What we need is legislation — and legislation now.

I would suggest a very simple Act making it *unlawful to fertilise an ovum taken from a woman save for the purpose of implanting that ovum in the woman from who it was taken so as to enable her to bear a child*. Some might criticise an Act in this form in that it does not restrict in vitro fertilisation to married couples. That is indeed a defect, but I do not think public opinion would accept such a restriction. In its favour the Act would outlaw womb leasing and ovum donation and thereby eliminate many of the legal problems and human tragedies I have mentioned. Finally, and above all, an Act of Parliament in this form would ensure that human life is brought into being solely, and only, in order that a baby may be born.

THE QUALITY OF LIFE

Mr Rex Brinkworth, MBE, BA, Cert. Ed. DCP, is the Director of the National Centre for Down's Syndrome, which he founded in 1970, and is run under the joint auspices of Down's Children Association and Birmingham Polytechnic. Mr Brinkworth is a trained teacher and psychologist and was, for twenty-two years, a specialist in retarded children in secondary schools.

6

THE QUALITY OF LIFE

MR REX BRINKWORTH

*The writer wishes to state that in this paper he is expresssing his
private views, both as a parent of two mentally handicapped
children and as the founder of the Down's Children's Association.
The views expressed do not necessarily represent those of Birmingham Polytechnic or of the Executive Committee of the Association,
which is officially neutral at present with regard to amniocentesis
and therapeutic abortion.*

When I began my work on Down's Syndrome, some 60 per cent
of our children were expected to die by the age of five and the
vast majority of those who did survive were severely or profoundly mentally handicapped. Today, I can say of our *treated*
children that some 3 per cent only have died over the past 17
years, and that far from being idiots, some 60 per cent today are,
or will be only mildly mentally handicapped, about 1 per cent
will fall within normal limits of intelligence, and the remainder
who are still within the ranks of the severely mentally handicapped are much less so in almost all cases than was expected in the
past. Today, some 80 per cent of Down's children live in the
community. When I was a child, probably 99% spent their lives
in institutions.

First, let me quote from the California Medical Journal for
September 1970. There it said: 'The relevance of each and every
human life has been the keystone of Western medicine, and is

the ethic which has caused physicians to try and preserve, protect, repair, prolong and enhance every human life. Since the old ethic has not been fully displaced, it has been necessary to separate the idea of abortion from the idea of killing which continues to be socially abhorrent. The result has been the curious avoidance of the scientific fact which everyone knows, that human life begins at conception and is continuous, whether intra or extra-uterine, until death.' To that view I subscribe, though my Association's Executive regards this as a contentious matter on which not all our members nor indeed all our Committee agree. Officially the Association remains neutral on abortion, though it states firmly that once born Down's children have the same right to life as do other children.

In this paper I put forward a rather wide view. It is conventional among paediatricians to describe the range of problems from early miscarriage and failure of implantation to the birth of severely handicapped children as 'the continuum of reproductive casualty'. I suggest that here has been, and is being developed, a more *sinister* continuum, ranging from the rejection of certain egg cells by medical specialists, through the abortion of the handicapped (and in many cases the healthy) to the elimination of handicapped children *after* birth, by a process which is euphemistically described as 'allowing the child to die'. I also propose to reflect on the hypothetical and the apparently real implications, not only for the handicapped, but potentially for us *all*, if we do not soberly consider the lessons of history and the trends of a modern and increasingly self-centred idea of life that in my view, threaten the whole of our civilisation, not only in the West, but also in the Eastern bloc.

Let us set out a formula:

(a) It is all right to select some egg cells for implantation in in vitro fertilisation, and to reject others, as eggs have no personality, nor can they feel pain if killed;

(b) It is all right to abort children who, for any reason, are not wanted;

(c) It may be regarded by some 23 per cent of the population (sampled by the Mori Poll of 1981 carried out by the BBC) to be all right to eliminate handicapped children after birth because they are a social burden on their families or on State financial resources.

In fact we have been here *before*! Less than fifty years ago in Nazi Germany, doctors co-operated with the State in liquidating many thousands of mentally, physically and psychiatrically affected children and adults. Those of you my age will know what ensued. Once the sanctity of life had been thus violated, once equipment had been assembled for large-scale murder, it was used by a totalitarian State to destroy successively those of whom the State disapproved for *other* reasons; trades unionists, churchmen, Jehovah's Witnesses, gypsies, and intellectuals who were perceived by the State as threatening or undesirable. Finally some six million Jews were liquidated.

Some may think it far-fetched to imagine any such thing could or would happen here, yet already we have travelled part of the path; already the medical body, both in Britain and Australia, has discussed whether old people might be painlessly killed at their own request, or when their dignity has been lost through senility. Already in Australia, Dr Chipman of the Department of Jurisprudence at the University of Sydney has been reported as saying: 'the unprecedented rise in the number of the elderly' and the 'enormous cost of caring for the aged in developed nations might cause the upcoming generation to call for "therapeutic" euthanasia'. He wrote this year in the Medical Post of Canada that (and I quote) '. . . the calculated killing of the elderly was not as absurd as it sounded . . . a generation which has readily accepted the idea of abortion as an efficient and morally neutral mechanism at the birth end will readily embrace . . . therapeutic euthanasia as a mechanism for disposing of a surplus population at the death end.' Press comment subsequently made the telling point — how ironic it would be if those now advocating the killing of the unborn by abortion would themselves be the ones killed by 'therapeutic euthanasia' should such a measure be adopted in the future.' I would add John Donne's famous phrase — 'Therefore do not ask for whom the bell tolls; it tolls for thee.' As a certain revolutionary once remarked — 'Gentlemen, we must hang together, otherwise you may be sure that we shall hang separately'.

To use a more flippant quotation to introduce my next reflections, I believe it was an American humorist who portrayed the leader of the Gadarene swine murmuring to his comrade as they ran over the cliff — 'I wonder how we were manoeuvred into this position'.

It may be that since the Second World War the rapid spread of communications has made us immune to the monotonous accounts in the press and other media of the murder, all over the world, of thousands and even millions of people every year by despotic or revolutionary regimes. Perhaps we have grown tolerant of such things, as we are apparently powerless to prevent them. It will, of course, be said that my comments on *our* possible future scenario are mere sensational alarmism, and that Britain has not been an autocracy for many centuries and never, since Cromwell, a dictatorship. Today, however, there are dangerous currents, which could very well at some future date make us, in turn, a totalitarian state, and Orwell foresaw such an eventuality in his book 1984, a year now only seven months ahead of us.

Slow and insidious process

The American Supreme Court led the legal way in the USA in 1973 saying that 'legal personhood does not exist prenatally', and many people around us today have also taken that first pernicious step towards the depersonalisation process that in Nazi Germany led to the acceptance, gradually, by the decent everyday German of horrors that he would never have contemplated had he not been subtly and crudely conditioned by propaganda. It is a slow and insidious process that conditions man to the idea that life is cheap. Already, up to this year, some 55 million foetuses have been aborted the world over. Even in 1975, the Population Crisis Committee in Washington said that 2 million abortions had taken place in Japan and in Brazil, one million each in the USA and Italy, and, according to an Indian Government Study that year, 3.8 millions had thus been eliminated in India, losses that over the years must have rivalled one of the World Wars. In 1979 the Committee reported some 40 million abortions, half of them illegal, had taken place, commenting that the incidence will rise with the desire for smaller families, lack of alternative family planning services and the growing number of women of child-bearing age. At the same time, the permissive society has resulted in a vast expansion of sexually transmitted diseases, some of them, like genital herpes type 2, presently incurable.

However, let us leave those figures to speak for themselves for the present. What do we mean by the term 'quality of life', of which such glib use is made today? Quality from whose point of view? The elite? The intelligent? The healthy? The doctors? The handicapped themselves? The Eugenics Society, which started in Britain in the 1880's with the aim of producing a race of supermen, an idea followed slavishly by Germany in the thirties? Should parents have the right to specify the child they want and reject him, terminally, if he or she happens to belong to the wrong sex, or may not be as intelligent or as healthy as his parents? I understand that already in the USA this is being considered, if not actually practised.

Should parents who wish to enjoy sex without responsibility be allowed to abort their offspring who might interfere with their selfish life-style so lavishly advertised as an ideal in many countries? Should those who are either too lazy, too careless, or too selfishly eager for the fullest sexual sensations to use efficient means of contraception be helped by the medical services when the woman becomes pregnant to dispose of her unwanted child? If these are to be answered in the affirmative, I would not give much for the future of human civilisation, whether in the East or the West.

When the American code of law changed from the old specification that abortion was only justified if the mother's life was in danger to a wider one which included psychological distresses and the defective foetus as additional justifications, it was said in Roe vs Wade that 'Maternity or additional offspring may force upon a woman a distressful life and future. Psychological harm may be eminent and physical life be taxed by health care. When there is distress for all concerned associated with the unwanted child and when there is a problem of bringing a child into the family, psychologically or otherwise unfit to care for it', abortion was justified. Did the courts imagine that such steps might reduce the number of unwanted and battered babies? Dr Edward Lenoski, Professor of Paediatrics at the University of Southern California, in a large survey, found that since the advent of abortion on demand, cruel infanticide, and child-battering increased three-fold, a logical result of the concept that life is cheap.

Do handicapped children break up the family? Well, first let us note that official figures state that in the Soviet Union, 30 per cent of marriages end in divorce. Japan averages a divorce every four minutes, in the USA about half of all marriages end in divorce, and in Britain, the number of divorce petitions rose fivefold between 1961 and 1981, and the present trend is toward a similar divorce rate to that of the USA. Was the causal factor a handicapped child in all these cases? No. It was the selfishness, immaturity and infidelity of one or both of the parties that lay behind such divorces among the 4000 families I serve, but so far only three mothers have said their divorce was mainly due to their husband's intolerance of their handicapped child. Certainly, others have been divorced, but the causes were rather those cited earlier, than was the presence of the handicapped child, and overall, as far as our records go, they show that the rate of divorce among our parents is substantially *lower* than the national average, as we teach both parents to join together in working productively towards the mental development of their child.

Views of the handicapped

What do the handicapped themselves think? We have not carried out a large survey on this, as many cannot express their views on such a subject yet, but I will say that the vast majority of our Down's children are happy more often than we are. My own daughter, who has Down's Syndrome, is among the more articulate and thoughtful and some of her comments over the years may well be relevant. Several years ago, she watched a programme on amniocentesis with great interest, and when it finished she turned to me and said simply 'They would have killed me'. Then turning anxiously to her mother she said, 'Mummy, are they going to kill me now?' What kind of a civilisation are we building where a child has to ask a question like that? Later, in 1981, she watched the famous case at Leicester Crown Court in the press and on television, and was bewildered by the verdict. It would be imprudent for me to comment on that case, no doubt, except to say that it must be thought curious that the jury was deliberately selected from people who had no knowledge or experience of handicap, that no expert on Down's Syndrome was called to give evidence (though several of us here today would have been willing to do so) and that when the son of one of our families who was present in the court asked one of the principal lawyers 'Why not?' — he muttered 'This case has nothing to do with Down's Syndrome' and turned his back. I am assured however by legal friends that the case did *not* set a legal precedent, as it was held in a Crown Court and did not go to Appeal in the Supreme Court.

However, one might ask how frequent such cases are. The interviewers in the programme 'Panorama' at that time said that they were not rare, especially in the case of spina bifida, where there were startling differences quoted for differential survival in different cities in the country. I can say that about eight years ago, I had personal experience of such an occurrence, but that I have been formally advised from various quarters not to make public what might appear as a controversial statement in the press and which could prove counterproductive in the fairly harmonious relationship of our Association with the medical body. I can merely say that such cases were not unknown a relatively few years ago, though whether they still occur and in what numbers, would be pure conjecture as they are not the subject of open discussion. My comment is not to be taken as a general statement of what may very well be the actions of a small minority of their profession.

You may ask why I did not report this matter at the time? I did in fact report it in confidence to another person, but was advised to say nothing which I could not find a means to verify, as I would receive no corroborative evidence from within the hospital, and might only make myself the defendant in a ruinous suit for slander against which my employers could not defend me. Hence I have otherwise remained silent on the matter to this day, as I cannot now remember at this distance of time (possibly by some repressive mechanism) which hospital was involved as I visited many at that time. But I have never forgotten that my silence effectively allowed a child to die, whom I might, albeit at great personal and professional risk, have saved. But you see, I was advised at the time that the professional code of confidentiality obliged me, as a visiting psychologist and a guest in the hospital, to disclose nothing that I had seen or heard concerning any doctor, nurse or patient in the course of my professional duties. The incident is unlikely in any event to recur in my experience, as on the course concerned, only those of my colleagues with nursing qualifications are now permitted into the hospitals as tutors to their students, possibly in the interests of professional security, as it was said at one point that the reason was that some of my colleagues had been overcome by some of the procedures and incidents that they had witnessed in the hospitals.

To revert to my earlier comments on the dangers of breaching the sanctity of life, however, it has been firmly indicated by demographic studies in Britain that by the year 2000, we shall have a very large aged population in relation to those who are still working, and that it will be difficult to finance the pensions and special care needed by the old. At the risk of being tedious,

I would repeat that there is a possibility, however unlikely and remote it may appear today, that if our society comes gradually to accept some of the negative views that have begun to prevail in recent years concerning the economic cost of the handicapped, the aged and the unborn child, we may ourselves be effectively signing a post-dated cheque to our own executioners when we reach old age, absurd though such nightmare fancies may appear at the present time.

As for the handicapped, it is true that their lives are relatively costly to the State, but I would remind everyone that they are someone's children, often very well loved by their families, and that a proper allocation of expenditure on research such as we carry out, as do other research and charitable bodies, would repay itself many times over if it helped to prevent the conception of children with certain major genetic errors, or to devise effective means, possibly by biochemical means as has already happened in the case of phenylketonuria and cretinism, to control the condition and remove its effects. I am reliably informed, notably at the Vatican Working Party in 1980 that the science of neo-natology, and the early diagnosis of fetal distress is already (though this is a new speciality) able to prevent handicapping conditions associated with blood imcompatibilities between mother and child, and if the work of Professor Smithells is proved correct by replicated studies, it might even be possible to eliminate spina bifida by adjustment of the diet of their mothers, though the sombre fact was expressed by Professor Mayor at the same working party that mental and physical handicaps taken on a world basis have as their largest single cause the malnutrition of parents in the Third World. Here again positive action by more favoured nations could go a long way towards eliminating these endemic causes of retardation.

I may be thought insensitive to the feelings of those who have to endure the most appalling handicaps, with which I am in fact all too familiar, or of those who have to care for them. Not at all. I know what intolerable agony is, having suffered it myself on a number of occasions in my own life, when I have been on the very edge of the grave. On one occasion, having suffered for days, the unspeakable agony of double dry pleurisy, I was given morphia and cocaine, which as you know are only normally given to those in extremis, for obvious reasons. Unable to see, speak or move, I could, however, still hear, as hearing is the last sense to go in the dying. I was quite aware of my situation, grateful for the relief of pain and unafraid of death. But I heard the doctor tell my mother that I could not see another dawn, and as Douglas Bader had done some fifteen years earlier, the statement awoke a characteristically stubborn sense of independence, and by refusing to sleep, a sleep from which I knew I would never awake, I survived to write this paper.

But never at any time would it have occurred to me that my doctors' duty extended further than the relief of pain. The idea that anyone should put another down like an injured racehorse is untenable as, though the Bible clearly gives Man dominion over the animals and *their* lives, it equally clearly denies Man the same right over that of other men, as Cain was the first to discover.

Nature takes its own course

My own father, three days before he died told me that he would like to discuss euthanasia with his doctors, as life had become utterly meaningless. For once I had to disagree. I told him that Nature itself would probably take its own course before long and that in any event, even in the unlikely event of his finding a compliant doctor, he would be not only giving up his own life, which perhaps one has some right to do at that stage, but would be compromising another human being at the Day of Judgement.

Moreover, having twice in my own family had to nurse a terminally ill, incoherent and doubly incontinent grandmother, I know the immense strain such care places on the family, as it does on many families with children more severely afflicted than are those with Down's Syndrome. But I still feel that any move to breach the sanctity of life, for however laudable a reason, as I see it, sets the deadly precedent of human selection, whose extension has infinite possibilities of evil.

It would be both impolite and irresponsible from the point of view of my employers and other bodies to comment further.

Finally, in the Panorama programme referred to earlier, one of our mothers gave a graphic account, which I still have on tape, of how her paediatrician tried to persuade her that she did not want her daughter, that Down's children commonly do not cry or feed well and tend to sleep their lives away, and further that if she did not, he could give her a small injection and she would sleep herself to death. But when that mother tried later to

63

swear an affidavit as to what had been said to her, no solicitor in that city could be induced to take it, and she eventually dropped the matter, partly out of fear, as her child was still on that paediatrican's list.

A month ago, I asked my daughter the same question that had been put to a spina bifida girl of fifteen in that programme, which we had just watched again, (we have never hidden the truth from my child and she has always been curious about her own condition, about which she knows a good deal more than most people do). The question was 'If you could go back to before you were born, knowing what you do now, would you rather we had let you live or die?' She paused and answered 'I would rather Mummy had a normal child'. 'But what would you have decided, Francoise', I asked again, 'to live or die?' 'To live of course', she replied. You may think me an insensitive father to ask my daughter such a question, but with us everything is open, and my daughter cheerfully accepts that she is handicapped and describes herself as such, though she says, 'I am not *mentally* handicapped, though. I'm just an ordinary slow learner.' She would rather not have Down's Syndrome of course, but as a stout Christian with a serene faith in God and a knowledge of the Bible at least as good as mine, she once said, 'I'm looking forward to the Resurrection. Then I'll be a normal girl, and I won't have Down's Syndrome.'

As for the quality of *her* life, she has left school and is perfectly competent to run a household in all respects, though I doubt whether she will ever cope completely independently with modern life with all its official forms, rates and taxes to think about. Others in her position may not be so lucky of course, and may, if we do not shortly aim to produce a good deal of sheltered accommodation within the community, end their days in hospital. We ourselves, and Francoise too, are all aware that she may age rapidly in middle life, and may (if we have not found the answer which with colleagues in France and Britain I am seeking) fall victim to Alzheimer's disease. Sensibly, however, she says that the Kingdom of God may well have come before then. Her quality of life is high and she is almost always happy. She is artistic, plays the piano tolerably to music, swims like a fish and has all her badges, reads and writes well enough and is sufficiently competent with numbers to manage her money properly. In fact, recently her elder sister who works in a bank, said she was a little envious of Francoise, as *she* already had a pension for life on leaving school while her elder sister had some forty years of hard work ahead of her before she should relax and spend her life in cultural pursuits as her sister can!

But, you may say, your child is an exception. Not exactly. Her IQ is only six points above that of the average Down's girl brought up by my methods. A vast number of others will do at least as well, and many will do very much better. Already over 40 of our children attend ordinary Infant and Junior schools, three are in Middle schools and four are in Secondary schools, three of them admittedly in remedial classes, but that does not imply a poor future. As the former Head of one of the largest Secondary Remedial Departments in the country, I can say that these children are of above average capacity, for my former classes, and that all my former pupils seem to have managed well enough since they left school. Until recently, I did not know of one who was unemployed, though of course, some may have become redundant since I last saw them.

What, however, of the really severely handicapped? I have known these too quite well and have seen many children with conditions that might make some of you faint, with distorted forms and features and no competence of any kind, speechless, blind, hydrocephalic, severely spastic or simply indescribable. One I know has spent the last fourteen years simply spinning round and round on the spot, staring at one raised finger, every single minute except when he is being fed or is asleep. Would not such children's quality of life be so poor that it would be merciful to kill them? No! For two good reasons. First, if you make the slightest breach in the dam that protects life, the flood will eventually pour through. Second, how can *we* judge what they feel? They may *appear* to feel nothing, either pleasure or pain, but as long as one lives and is conscious, the brain is registering something, and we cannot and should not presume to guess at what they themselves perceive as pleasure or pain.

Ten years ago, I visited a very severely spastic man in a well known and excellent hospital. He has never been able to feed himself, wash or toilet himself, or to speak, but years ago an inspired Charge Nurse taught him to read and write using a typewriter with one toe, the only part of his body he can control. I was accompanied by a colleague who had nursed this man years before and knew him well enough to ask what, to an outsider, might have seemed an insensitive question, as that which I earlier mentioned as having addressed to my daughter.

65

'Tell me Bill,' he asked, 'does your condition ever bug you?' Bill gave his equivalent of a grin and typed laboriously back 'no, but it bugs other people!' Then, when my student had left the room, he started to write again with his foot, this time to me, a stranger. He wrote - 'I'm me. I've been me all my life. I know what it is like to be me. I don't know what it's like to be you, so how can you know what it's like to be me?' A good question, and one on which we ought to ponder before making judgements about other people's lives, based on our own experience and feelings. If the handicapped are well and properly looked after, they are not, in my experience any more unhappy than most of us; if they are in pain, it can be relieved as a rule. They do not have a monopoly on pain. It is something most of us share at some time. I do, for internal reasons, most of the time.

Research and selection

What then of the subject of this conference? I know a certain amount about human genetics so I can say that any form of research using human eggs and spermatozoa presents major moral problems, simply because it involves the perilous principle of *selection* from which so many more evils can follow and do follow. A rejected egg may not feel pain, but it was a potential human being, with all its message mysteriously coiled up within it. Even before conception, we are, to some degree, potential individuals, different from our mother, in that our chromosomes have already exchanged parts of their message at first meiosis. But of course, we cannot develop if our father does not provide the other half of the message necessary to trigger off our development into a human being. Once fertilised however, we are already a fully potential person. No-one at that stage can, without exceptional circumstances, predict the future of that egg. Granted that, as many geneticists point out in justifications of their actions, nature itself eliminates a vast proportion of the children we conceive. Some put the rate of miscarriage from very early failure of implantation to late miscarriage and natural abortion as high as between one in seven and one in two of all fertilised eggs! That, however, is in the hands of God. For us to intervene with further selection processes seems to me not only perilous but unchristian and unjewish too, if we consider Exodus Chapter 21, verses 22 and 23 where it says, 'If men strive and hurt a woman with child so that her fruit depart from her and yet no mischief follow, he shall be surely punished according as the woman's husband will lay on him and he shall pay as the judges determine. And if any mischief follow (which scholars interpret to mean if either the woman or the child are harmed) THEN THOU SHALT GIVE LIFE FOR LIFE'.

I would now like to examine in a personal way the motivations of a scientist and act to a degree as Devil's Advocate. I daresay that some at least of you here have an interest in human biology and, like myself, are keen microscopists. Like myself perhaps, you commonly borrow some of your own cells for microscopical study. Generally, we either use blood cells which are quite easy to obtain and not difficult in the case of leucocytes to keep alive for quite a while outside the body to which they belonged. I also quite commonly use cells from inside my cheek which are not so painful to obtain as blood samples are. I have often examined my own cells thus, though I have not the skills or equipment to get them to undergo mitotic divisions. But I often think, a short while ago that cell was part of me and under the control of my brain, biological and nervous systems and probably some form of intercellular communication, an area in which there are still many mysteries. Who is it, or who are they now? They are still alive but no longer in a sense me. It is a very thought provoking thing to do. I also have a number of dead and stained specimens of human ovaries and testes, and in one of them I had the unusual chance of finding one undergoing at the time of its removal a genetic division. The chromosomes are clearly visible there.

Now if I had the skills and equipment of doctors such as Steptoe and Edwards, I might, I can very well imagine, try to meddle with that life in my hands in view of the normal human propensity for curiosity and the pursuit of knowledge and less admirable but thoroughly human desire for scientific glory and academic recognition. I would argue that out of the body the cells are no longer their original owner's possession, and that to fertilise an egg with the husband's sperm at least is not materially different from letting the parents do that in the usual way of nature, something that because of some fault in the reproductive organs they cannot do for themselves. I might well argue that that was legitimate, though I would not myself countenance the use of artificial insemination by an unknown donor, because to me that would be the equivalent of adultery, or even on a rare possibility if pooled samples of sperm were used, even incest, though the physical act would be missing. One can therefore imagine what temptations lie with those scientists who have both the knowledge and equipment to carry out in vitro fertilisation; and one cannot easily say how, in their position, one would rationalise one's action. But, it would probably be that they were helping people who cannot have children through some fault of nature which they are innocent of. The crux of the matter however is the element of selection. Either I throw away some of my own cells having examined them under phase-contrast microscopy or I keep a few for fixing and staining for later study. But the cells I use are not my reproductive cells; and I do not, in any event, meddle with them apart from the technical processes of fixing and staining them.

However, to put a second case. For the past seventeen years beginning with my own daughter, I have carried out extensive work aimed at changing children with Down's Syndrome by various means into something nearer to our own normal form and function. Not only do I alter the efficiency of their nervous systems by using special methods of stimulation early in life, but I even change by a process that I myself do not fully understand, their physical appearance and structure to such a degree that in a few cases the signs of their condition, apart from a short stature, are no longer present, and in most cases, at least much less evident. Now you could, as one of our more devout Irish members once put it to me, argue that I too am meddling with what God has made and am changing it to something which the child's parents want. I have thought about this many times, but have concluded that God did not intend children to be born with handicaps any more than he originally wished us to suffer from crippling and agonising diseases. If it is legitimate to attack our enemies in the form of bacteria and viruses it would then appear legitimate to alter people for their own benefit, something which after all a teacher tries to do every day of his life in other ways.

But the essential error in logic, as I see it, is that we forget what humans in a position of power generally do with their powers. I have noted that at times academics can be as unscrupulous as anyone in their desire to obtain a result and to be the first to publish. All of us are under that sort of pressure, and I am no exception. It is also common experience that if one man can devise a technique beneficial to mankind, some other person, or even the same person, being like the rest of us a human being and a sinner, may turn that power to evil ends, as

Man almost invariably does. A knife can serve to cut our beef or to murder our neighbour. Power over human reproduction is an awesome one with unlimited opportunities for evil in producing hybrid creatures or in selective reproduction outside the laws of God on that specific subject. One could, for example, in a totalitarian state choose to breed people like racehorses to produce varieties like H. G. Wells's Eloi and Morlocks to form a society with an elite and a rate of slaves or mindless and brutal soldiery for use in wars. Already, I understand in one part of the world, scientists are engaged in modifying the responses of soldiers' nervous systems to produce fearless troops who might be well-nigh invincible.

Changed person

Even in my own work I have deliberately, though through natural means, changed my own child from what she was as a baby, a very poor specimen of Down's Syndrome, into a quite different person today. Doubtless the reproductive scientists would put up the same argument. There is however a difference. I may have selected for my child those behaviours which I felt would be most beneficial to her, but I would not, even if I had had the chance, have aborted her simply because she had Down's Syndrome as some would do. Nor would my wife. It is too late for us now to have further children; but if by some miracle we did conceive another child at our age, when the risk of Down's Syndrome is as high as 1 in 12, we still would not seek amniocentesis as we would not in any event abort our child. We would simply start all over again, probably with more success given the amount I have learned during the seventeen years of my daughter's life. I think therefore that above all things, we should regard in vitro fertilisation with great reserve since as I have said earlier, selection of people to live or die at any stage of their existence means putting ourselves in the place of God; in which case I have no doubt that He will eventually call us to account for the same sins of pride and want of power that turned Lucifer into Satan, the adversary. What that might lead to I have already, I hope, set out as a logical and probable progression.

Even in my own published work about my daughter and thousands of other Down's babies I still do not and will not report a very few of the things I did in her early days of life as some of them could easily be taken up by other scientists for potentially evil ends. Those few secrets I feel I should take with me to the grave.

With the lessons of human history and of current human conduct we cannot, and should not, come to the blasphemous belief that Man is capable of producing a Brave New World, except one of the kind forecast by Huxley. My hope is not in that sort of world, but ultimately in the Kingdom of God. Then too, I have in mind that God said in Genesis when Adam had eaten of the fruit of the tree of knowledge, 'Behold, the man is become as one of us to know good and evil and now lest he put forth his hand and take also of the tree of life and eat and live for ever, therefore the Lord God sent him forth from the garden of Eden to till the ground from when he was taken.' Geneticists may claim that they may find the causes of mental and physical handicaps if they are allowed to experiment with human cells; but having in mind man's insatiable curiosity, evil nature, and lust for power as much as knowledge, I would foresee them looking next for the secret of life itself, that is, to eat at last of the fruit of the tree of life! I am sufficiently fundamental in my faith to believe that God will choose his time to end this world before we destroy it ourselves, as we can already do a thousand times over with our nuclear weapons, or before we presume upon his sole prerogative, that of creating life itself.

Instead of the cowardly flight before handicapping conditions that at least a proportion of the doctors I know are currently making, let us rather seek energetically the causes of these handicaps, and attempt at least either to prevent or to cure them, though not through in vitro fertilisation, in which much danger lies. I have already been privileged to help thousands of Down's children to develop far better than they did in the past, though I cannot cure their condition. I believe, however, on the basis of current knowledge and new technique, that we *could* discover these things, perhaps within a decade, if we were given even a fraction of the money spent each day on armaments designed to kill and maim millions. We *must* escape from the ancient philosophy that if you cannot cure the disease you kill the patient. This prevailed during the Plague.

NOTE

Professor Sir William Liley, pioneer of neonatology and the inventor of amniocentesis, wrote:

> Biologically at no stage can we subscribe to the view that the foetus is a mere appendage of the mother; mother and baby are separate individuals from conception . . .
>
> You would think the knowledge would bring a new respect for the unborn. Instead, some are hell-bent on his destruction — just when he has achieved physical and emotional maturity . . .
>
> The unborn are small, defenceless, nameless and voiceless. He has not yet reached the age of social significance and he cannot strike back for himself . . .'

Sir William's aim was really not to abort children, but to identify them in the womb, diagnose their condition and if possible, *treat* them in utero. When in Rome in 1980 he gave the writer the impression that he was dismayed at the use which has since been made of his invention of the technique. He was a close friend of Professor Lejeune, an ardent opponent of abortion on any grounds other than a real risk to the mother's life, and was the New Zealand delegate at the Vatican Conference of 1980 where eight leading authorities (including the writer) reported to the Pope advances in a variety of fields of handicap. It might be noted, as an expression of Sir William's views, that he and his wife adopted a Down's Syndrome girl some years ago which is not the act of a man who would favour the prenatal elimination of such children.

R.B.

SOCIAL AND ETHICAL ASPECTS OF IVF

Dr Teresa Iglesias is Research Officer at The Linacre Centre, an institute for the study of the ethics of health care. She obtained her primary degree in Philosophy at Madrid University, and a Doctorate in Philosophy at Oxford. She was previously a lecturer in Philosophy at University College, Dublin, and held a visiting fellowship at New Hall, Cambridge.

7
SOCIAL AND ETHICAL ASPECTS OF IVF

DR TERESA IGLESIAS

Setting the Scene: Central Questions and Problems

One of the most important decisions that our government will have to make in the near future is concerned with the *legal status* of the human embryo[1]. The government's future decision, as well as the resolution of the *basic social* and *ethical* issues raised by the practice of human in vitro fertilization (IVF), will depend, if it is reasonably and fairly made, on the *moral status* of the human embryo. That is to say, everything will turn on the answer we give to this question: What kind of respect is due to the human embryo? Is the human embryo to be protected as a human being, or as a property? Legal and public policy issues are not independent of moral evaluations nor of facts: they ultimately rest upon them.

The recognition of facts and the moral evaluations we make to answer this question will be of enormous significance, not only for the life of this nation, but also for the world at large. The human family is, at this stage of history, already bound and knitted together as a whole. Not only economic and nuclear policies, but also policies regarding health and biomedical research adopted by countries with technical and industrial resources, like this one, will eventually affect millions of human beings, for good or ill. Our responsibilities for our fellow human beings are no longer national, they are now of world wide character, affecting the human family as a whole. Every personal and social decision sets a standard. By such decisions we construct the moral climate of our world. Britain has been a pioneer in the technique of IVF; the moral and legal stand this country takes now, concerning the aims and procedures of this technique, will be inevitably of pioneering significance for the world at large as well. Britain cannot ignore this responsibility or be blind to it.

Let me introduce what seem to me to be the three most fundamental ethical issues related to the aims and procedures of IVF programmes, namely, (a) the question of the 'spare' embryos in the IVF and embryo replacement (ER) programme; (b) the still experimental character of this programme; and (c) the direct experimentation on human embryos for scientific purposes. We shall later consider some of the social implications of these issues. I shall begin by referring briefly to Dr R G Edwards' own formulation of the problems, and to his ethical opinions, not only because he has from the beginning presented them openly for discussion but also because these opinions are quite representative of most of his colleagues' researches in the field, and thus in their programmes they bear a considerable weight[2].

Fourteen years ago, in 1969, Dr R G Edwards identified some of the medical and scientific possibilities attached to the study of and experiments with human embryos which he and others were beginning to engage in then[3]. They were: the alleviation of human infertility; the development of knowledge of contraceptive means (envisaging even a situation where medical ways could be found to "immunise" people against fertilization or implantation)[4]; alleviation of genetic diseases and deformities and of other forms of diseases; and further development of the knowledge of human reproduction and of embryology in general.

(a) *The 'spare' embryos*. For Dr Edwards the basic ethical question in connection with the therapeutic aim of IVF and embryo replacement to alleviate human infertility was seen as early as 1969 in these terms: 'We would have to take several eggs from the mother, and transfer only one or two back into her. The remainder would be thrown away. Is it acceptable to discard the excess embryos?'[5] This question is still with us. It is important to note that it was taken then, and is still taken now, as a fundamental *ethical* question. This is so because we are implicitly recognising that the embryo we are dealing with is *human* in a particular way, i.e. it is not a mere 'human tissue', a 'cluster of cells', or a 'speck of matter'. If that were all the human embryo was, the question would be altogether irrelevant; a mere speck of human tissue, even the highly organised unfertilized egg itself, could not raise such a fundamental ethical question.

The ethical acceptability of discarding embryos, or, as an alternative, of freezing them, is given a variety of justifications at present — as we shall later see; but perhaps at the root of all justifications lies the one that Dr Edwards gave in 1969: '. . . by throwing the excess embryos away, we are doing no more than any couple using the intra-uterine device for contraception . . . In a society which sanctions the abortion of a fully-formed fetus, the discarding of such a minute, undifferentiated embryo should be acceptable to most people'[6]. Indeed this is the case. But we know that acceptability by most people does not make a practice morally right — counting heads is not a way to determine what is good or evil[7]. We know, however, that a socialised practice does indeed change our moral attitudes, even if the change is not morally for the 'better'. We are all exposed and vulnerable in this respect.

(b) *The experimental character of IVF and embryo replacement.* This question has not been raised as ethical by those directly involved in the IVF programmes but by others[8], both in its early stages and at present. It is true that the current situation as regards IVF differs greatly from the early one in its *achievements*, which have been attained after 'the lonely and frustrating pathway that ultimately led to the joy of the birth of Louise Brown'[9], to use Dr Edwards' own words. Yet the ethical issues remain with us, and some more acutely so because of the advances. Despite the advances, many scientific uncertainties still prevail[10], showing that this form of human generation entails serious risks, particularly for the child-to-be. Dr Edwards holds, with other researchers, that because the 'evidence of the liveborn children confirms observations in animals that the culture of preimplantation embryos *in vitro* is safe and imposes no extra risks on the child . . . the procedure could be introduced into clinical medicine with very few reservations, especially with the back-up screening provided by ultrasonic scans, amniocentesis and other tests in later pregnancy'[11]. It is indicative that despite the optimism, the reservations are still there (the more so since the practice of freezing the spare embryos is now used[12]). The 'back-up' procedures must be viewed in the light of their ultimate *aims*. It must also be noted that it is normal practice in IVF-ER programmes not to implant the newly fertilized embryo if it is developing abnormally[13]. In view of this fact alone the moral acceptability of any IVF therapeutic programme may be questioned, as we shall see later.

(c) *Experimenting with human embryos and the study of embryology*. In 1981 in Cambridge the first 'Bourn Hall' meeting of international character took place. It gathered authorities on IVF from this country, Switzerland, West Germany, Sweden, Australia, USA, France and Austria[14]. It was there that the real possibility was acknowledged of growing embryos *in vitro* up to the stage where the early beginnings of organic differentiation occur: 'analyses on differentiation and early organogenesis in the human embryo are now feasible'[15]. Dr Edwards also pointed out: "Better methods may be devised for culturing embryos *in vitro*, and the nature of normal and abnormal growth could be analysed. Methods might be introduced to use embryonic tissues for the cellular repair of damaged tissues in adults, especially for organs without renewal of stem cells"[16]. Will these methods and aims be ethically acceptable? —Dr Edwards asks. The answer he gives now is the same as the one given in 1969, and the reason for his unchanged moral stance is the same: 'The ethical issues involved in establishing and studying early embryos *in vitro* should be acceptable in view of the potential advantages of this work. These issues seem to be minor in relation to other ethical dilemmas involving embryos and fetuses e.g. the accepted and widespread use of I.U.D.s and abortion for family limitation'[17]. The central ethical question raised by the scientific interest of the IVF programme was put by Dr Edwards to his colleagues at the Bourn Hall Symposium in these terms: 'We have to make a decision as to whether human embryology should be pursued for its own sake'[18].

Because the decisions to be taken are moral and social in character they affect us all. The need for cooperative dialogue, weighty and truthful consideration of the facts, as well as unswerving personal commitment to moral integrity, are necessary ingredients — although rare virtues — at a time when such crucial decisions are to be made.

What routes may we take to come to such decisions? How are the aims and procedures, the means and ends, of IVF, and of the study of embryology, to be assessed?

I propose to take two complementary routes which appear

inevitable: one moral in character, the other biological. The first route hinges on a consideration of the value of human life, the second on a biological consideration of the human being. These two routes will lead us to the cross-road of the moral status of the human embryo, where a fundamental option of moral character will have to be made by each one of us, and by the law, and so by society as a whole. The forms of social life, related to the human reproduction which will be promoted and allowed to develop, will primarily depend on this fundamental option. Obviously, this option is itself dependent on the attitudes and capacities embedded in our modes of thinking and living which enable us to recognise (or hinder us from recognising) true moral values.

I. A moral evaluation: 'no human being is a property'

Central to our moral decisions and judgements is our basic moral vision i.e. the moral perspective in which we stand. Part of this vision is our attitude towards human life i.e. the way we regard and value our fellow human beings. Talk of our commitment to 'humanity', to its overall good and progress, necessarily takes the concrete form of a commitment to, or a disregard for, this or that individual human being. Thus our personal moral attitude could be summed up as 'what we would be prepared to do, or in fact do, to any individual human being — including ourselves'.

A particular moral vision and an attitude towards human life could be expressed in this principle: 'no human being is a property'. A look back into social history can illustrate in slavery the origins and content of this principle. Historically, slavery was a social institutionalisation of regarding certain human beings as properties of others, and treating them as such. A slave was his master's property. He had no claim over his life and liberty. He was instrumental, and so could be used, exploited, or even killed. A slave was radically a means to the interests and benefits of his master.

The abolition of slavery is one of the greatest steps in the moral development of the human family. It has seen its legal realisation in our present time. This abolition became the social expression of recognition of the fundamental equality of all human beings, as having an inviolable status as regards life and liberty.

Thus, human beings are not properties, objects, or instruments of use to serve the benefits and interests of others. 'No human being is a property' is a moral premise of our contemporary society which expresses an egalitarian vision of man, attained through long social struggle and by the suffering lives and deaths of many individual human beings. It has been perhaps the most powerful moral idea — and ideal — at work in the world for the last two centuries, and still is so in the present[19]. Recognising the radical equality of status of all members of the human family leads us also to recognise what might be meant by the principle 'respect for persons'. This respect is a fundamental requirement of justice, in virtue of which no human being is to be used or exploited for any purpose whatsoever. It is a recognition that *every human being has at least the right not to be used merely as a means to the needs or interests of others and every harmless human being has at least the right not to be killed*[20]. 'Not to be used, not to be killed', is the ultimate moral ground where the roots of justice lie, and so it is the point of departure for our dealings with one another in all the social contexts and social forms of life in which we find ourselves and which we continuously create. Recognition of these basic rights amounts to an ultimate moral obligation for those of us who *can* actually use or actually kill others.

This recognition pervades our international declarations and national bills of rights. It was in 1948 that for the first time in history many countries of the world united in a *Universal Declaration of Human Rights*. Here they officially acknowledged the fundamental moral equality of 'all members of the human family' (Preamble); 'the right to life and liberty' of each one of them (Art.3); the prohibition of all forms of slavery (Art.4); and the demand to 'act towards one another in a spirit of brotherhood' (Art.1).

This same moral vision is enshrined in our law, which is designed to guarantee and protect the inviolable status of every individual human being. We are all equal before the law because we are of equal standing as members of the human family.

The paramount and inviolable value of the individual human being has also been part of the moral vision that the medical profession in its attempt to serve life has expressed in its codes of practice. The most ancient one we possess, *The Hippocratic Code*, sets 'the beginning of medical ethics'[21] in the principle 'primum non nocere'. The code says: 'I will keep the sick from harm and injustice'. Not to harm, not to commit injustice, minimally involves not to use or damage anyone in the most radical way — i.e. not to destroy or kill anyone.

The World Medical Association, in the *Declaration of Helsinki* (dating from 1964 and revised in 1975), which is concerned with recommendations to doctors in biomedical research involving human subjects, adopts the same attitude towards respect for the life of the individual human being. The Declaration states: 'Concern for the interests of the subject must always prevail over the interest of science and society'[22].

The final words of the Declaration are: 'In research on man, the interest of science and society should never take precedence over considerations related to the well-being of the subject'[23].

It is not only that the historical social struggle for the abolition of slavery and racialism, our declarations and bills of rights, the law, and medical codes of practice, bear witness to the paramount value of the individual human being; in fact, the recognition of this value, and the moral demand to act in accordance with it, constitutes a corner stone or 'first principle' of traditional moral philosophies. Never treat a human being as a mere means, but always as an end, said Kant.

The religious moral thinking of the jewish-christian tradition has lived, and lives, with this same moral vision: 'love your neighbour' is a first commandment. By 'neighbour' is understood any human being; by 'love', the measure of respect, care and responsibility for another which is not only incapable of committing any injustice against him, but is even capable of generating the strength to give one's own life for him.

It must be recalled, though, that for the utilitarian tradition in philosophy (much adopted in this country in principle and in practice) respect for the individual human being is not the paramount moral value; the paramount moral value is rather 'the greatest good for the greatest number'. This allows that, given certain circumstances, the life or lives of individual human beings may be regarded as instrumental, and so expendable, for that 'greater good'. Ultimately, in utilitarianism, all values can be 'traded off'; human beings themselves can be[24]. This is not so for the non-utilitarian outlook I have been presenting, and to which I adhere. Within this latter outlook any weighing and comparing of values occurs only on the presupposition that respect for the inviolability of each individual human being is under no circumstances to be 'traded off'

81

i.e. the direct destruction of innocent human life is never regarded as justifiable.

II. Who counts as a human being?

Who counts as a member of the human family? Who counts as a human being? These questions could be asked from two different perspectives: the biological and the moral. In biological terms the question would mean: who counts as a member of the human species? When does such a member come into existence? In moral terms the question would mean: who are we to regard as enjoying a human moral status with inviolability of life? Who is to be respected as one of us?

The biological question and the moral question are different. Yet they are closely related, both historically and at present. Historically, denial of human moral status to a group of human beings by another group — or the claim that they were 'less human' — has ultimately been based upon, or justified in terms of, organic or biological differences: these lesser human beings were different because of the colour of their skin, because they were female, because they were children, etc. Also, the fact that a human being was born into a particular social class or status e.g. as a slave or as an untouchable, was not regarded as merely a matter of convention but rather as something which might be written into one's own being by nature. Even for Aristotle nature, which made a human being a man or a woman, made some human beings slaves.

Present scientific and medical developments in life-saving and reproductive techniques and in genetics, as well as the issues of abortion and contraception, have brought the question 'who counts as a human being?' to the fore both in its biological and in its moral dimensions. It was only a year ago that a flurry of concern was expressed about experimentation with human embryos in this country, in which this question was central. The media in all its forms conveyed the stir. A common opinion then expressed was this: (I take it only as representative of the hundreds of others expressed in similar terms) "We lack any common basis for resolving the ethical issues of what can be done to the embryo. These turn on the question of when human life begins"[(25)]. It appears that the moral and biological questions are taken to be related here. The reasoning behind the claim seems to be this: since biologically it is not certain when a human being comes into existence, or when a human life begins, we cannot easily resolve when the moral status of respect and protection is to be given to a human embryo. We do not really know if a human embryo *is* a human being. Thus the decision when to treat it with respect — or when it would be wrong to kill it — must be arbitrary to a certain extent. If we knew for certain when a human being came into existence, we would recognise *then* his human moral status.

Is this really the case? Perhaps for many of us it is, but it has not been the line of thought taken, for example, by the Ethics Committee of the Royal College of Obstetricians and Gynaecologists in their recent *Report on in Vitro Fertilisation and Embryo Replacement or Transfer* of March 1983. The Report notes: 'The question 'when does life begin?' is a physical question, not a moral one . . .' (Sec. 13.4) — I presume that by 'physical' they mean 'biological'. The Report states: 'The proper moral question is not 'when does life begin?' but 'at what point in the development of the embryo do we attribute to it the protection due to a human being?' (Sec. 13.5).

It is indeed right to recognise that 'when does life begin?' is *not* a moral question and distinct from the question of the recognition of the protection due to a human being. Yet recognition of the respect due to a human being requires as a necessary condition that one know who *is* a human being. The fact that these two questions are distinct from each other — which indeed they are — means, for the Ethics Committee of the RCOG, that the biological definition of a human being, as a member of the human species whose existence begins at conception, does not settle the question as to which human beings enjoy moral status. In fact they claim that the use and destruction of the human embryo for purposes of biomedical research should not be prohibited. The general principle behind this thinking is: to belong to the human species does not guarantee human moral status.

This has not been the principle adopted by other bodies[26] e.g. the Royal College of General Practitioners in their Report on IVF to the Warnock Committee. Although the RCGP Report as a whole lacks moral consistency, it claims: 'Although there are conflicting views about the onset of human life, the process can be considered to commence at fertilization since this is the point at which a genetically complete embryo is formed. From that moment therefore, the embryo should be treated with respect, and experimentation on human embryos should be subject to the same ethical considerations as on children and adults'[27]. If we are to judge solely from this statement, the position here adopted is this: the biological definition of a human being as a new complete organism in the species 'human', constitutes the basis for recognising that the embryo has human moral status similar to that attributed to other human beings — like children and adults.

Even if we take this mode of reasoning to be correct, it must be accepted, of course, that scientific facts, e.g. biological facts such as the determination of the beginning of a human being, do not and cannot by themselves determine our moral attitudes and our moral evaluations. These have their roots in our *moral* beings i.e. in our consciences and modes of judging and living, in our ultimate visions of the value of others, of reality and of God. These, indeed, science cannot determine. So we must be grateful for having been reminded by the RCOG's Report of the difference there is between the scientific and the moral order. Yet to invoke such a difference of orders, as well as to invoke the Western moral tradition 'grounded in Aristotelian thought and science' to substantiate their claim that the embryo need not be given a human moral status from its beginning, is not justified. The Report says: 'the attribution of absolute protection to the human embryo from its earliest beginning has no long history in Western moral tradition . . . the tradition grounded in Aristotelian thought and science . . .' (Sec. 13.5). Indeed this is not the case. It can be shown that in that tradition the biological question has been inseparable from the moral question at least in these two important respects: (a) in the recognition that there was a *biological process of generation* with a beginning which would ultimately develop into a human being, and (b) in the determination as to when in that process the embryo attained *full biological humanity* and, hence, could be considered a human being with full moral status. These considerations were *decisive* for what was to be regarded as morally permissible and in determining penal sanctions.

Let me go back in history for a moment to illustrate this. We may remember that a doctrine of delayed animation was held over a number of centuries and by many christian thinkers, following Aristotle. This doctrine maintained that the fetus only at a certain stage of its development attains 'humanity' i.e. becomes a member of the species 'human', becomes 'homo'. It is important to note that this belief about the time of animation was *never* looked on as a *moral* dividing line between permissible and impermissible abortion i.e. direct destruction of nascent life. Abortion was always wrong. Even if there was no certainty that the embryo was human at conception the fact that, at that moment, the biological process of generation of what was to become a new human being had started was sufficient reason to consider that it was immoral to directly attempt the destruction of such nascent life[28]. In this respect current debate and attitudes are departing notably from the past tradition rather than being suppported by it.

The belief in delayed animation played a role in the *penal* and *penitential* practices of the Church i.e. in relation to the status that a person had within the christian community after committing that *crime*, and whether or not the crime was regarded as homicide or murder (even if the child was unborn). Thus the embryo, which it was known would develop into the adult human being, always enjoyed protection of life from its early beginnings, independently of the belief in delayed animation; to attempt to destroy it directly was to kill nascent human life, for which there never was considered to be moral justification[29]. And when the fetus was regarded as having full humanity, to destroy him or her was to commit the crime of murder.

It is important to ask ourselves why the belief in delayed animation was held by Aristotle and the Aristotelians who followed after him. And the answer can be found in the biological knowledge they had concerning generation. Their belief rested primarily on a biological premise, namely, that there was no *human life* at all in the early stages of the life of the embryo. The embryo's life was of an undifferentiated, non-specific, kind: first vegetative and then animal[30]. This non-differentiation applied to embryos of human kind and of non-human kind. There was held to be generic but not specific differentiation in the early beginnings of life. The embryo is an animal before it is a human being, affirmed Aristotle, and this was repeated by Aquinas[31]. So merely animal life had to be transformed into human life (i.e. a *substantial change* had to occur) extrinsically by the principle of human life — the human soul[32]. This principle of life accounted for the unity, organisation, and intrinsic development of the new human being, as *human* being.

It was not then known that the embryo was from the beginning an *organised*, *unique*, living *unity* with *intrinsic capacity for development* from the beginning of its existence into the adult human organism; or, second, that this well-unified and organised entity was *human in character from its beginning* and nothing but human, given its material unity and organisation, and its specific kind of life. If 'humanity' could not be detected in the material biological unity and organisation of the embryo, was it not reasonable to invoke a principle to account for it? But if it is there from the beginning, why should such a principle be invoked?

It can reasonably be argued that if Aristotle and his followers had had the biological knowledge we possess today, they would have had to claim, in virtue of the principles they held about matter and form, that the *substantial change* that occurs when generative human material becomes a human being must occur at fertilization and not at any other later stage. For it is at fertilization that a being of human material unity, organisation, and constant dynamism of intrinsic self-development of a human kind — and only of a human kind — comes into existence. The soul, the principle of life, the 'anima' is the form of the human organism from its beginning, i.e. it makes it what it *is*: giving it existence, a new living human organism, a new member of the human species. It is clear that Aristotle could not ascribe human moral status to a being which in his opinion was not biologically human.

The biological sciences can tell us today that a new human being, a new member of the human species, comes into existence at fertilization. I trust the scientists in taking the following claims as a matter of scientific evidence. The cell is at once the universal component of all living bodies and the factor that unites one generation to the next. The human body is constituted by two kinds of cells: the somatic and the generative. The first kind contain 46 chromosomes — the number of chromosomes proper to the human species. The generative cells contain half the 46 chromosomes: 23. The ovum and the sperm are cells of the latter kind, the ones capable of establishing the link between one human generation and the next. They are the cells bringing about human reproduction. When an ovum and a sperm unite and their pro-nuclei fuse, a new single cell comes into being, the most remarkable of all cells. Its coming into existence reveals both the baffling mystery and the comprehensibility of human life. Let me quote François Jacob's vision of this cell:

> 'The formation of a man from an egg is a marvel of exactitude and precision. How can millions of millions of cells emerge, in specialised lineages, in perfect order in time and space, from a single cell? This baffles the imagination. During embryonic development, the instructions contained in the chromosomes of the egg are gradually translated and executed, determining when and where the thousands of molecular species that constitute the body of an adult are to be formed. The whole plan of growth, the whole series of operations to be carried out, the order and the site of syntheses and their coordination are all written down in the nucleic-acid message. And in the execution of the plan, there are few failures: the accuracy of the system may be measured by the rarity of abortions and monsters'[33],

By considering the differences and similarities between the individual cells, the ovum, the sperm, and the zygote they bring about, very significant facts emerge. One is connected with the question: when does human life begin? A biologist has answered the question thus: 'Never. Life ends often, but it never begins. It is just passed on from one cell to another. All biologists . . . are in agreement on that answer'[34].

Indeed, not only life but humanity is a continuum. For an ovum must be a live cell and a human cell (and mature) to be fertilized by a sperm, which must also be alive and human to bring about a new living human cell: the zygote. Their 'specific' humanity and life they have received from other cells. Thus the question, when does human life begin, must strictly be answered: it does not begin, it is continuous, it is transmitted.

It is important to note that life only exists in *individuals of specific forms*, i.e. it only exists and is communicated in and through the individual organisms that constitute the members of this or that species. This is a fact. So a legitimate question arises: *when does human life become a human being?* When does a new human organism, a new item in the species, come into existence? The biological sciences have answered this question in a definite way: at fertilization, neither before nor after[35]. At fertilization a new, unique, complete human organism begins. It is human like all the other cells, but its humanity differs in *kind* from that of other cells. Biologists have put it this way:

87

'A zygote is human because within its total DNA conformation are the DNA structures which determine, and are common to, the human species. It is a specific human being because the total DNA conformation of this individual is constant at all points of the organism's existence.'[36]

So it is not true to say that 'Everything that can be said about the potential of the embryo can also be said of the potential of the egg and sperm'[37]. First, the genetic constitution of the zygote is not that of the egg and sperm. The 46 chromosomes in the zygote are a new kind of reality from the 23 in the sperm and the ovum added quantitatively. Second, the zygote is from the beginning a genetically complete, organised, unique individual organism in the species. If it does not die and is not killed, it will develop into a man or a woman. This is not the destiny of ovum and sperm if they do not unite. Third, the development and its finality is inbuilt in the power of the new organism itself; this development may be described 'as a process of becoming the one he already is'[38]. That is why I can truly say that my life as an adult is continuous with my life as a child, and my life as a zygote. I am trillions of cells now, but once I began as a single cell, a zygote. Yet I have never been an unfertilized ovum, nor a sperm. The beginning of me, mysteriously so indeed, must be traced back to fertilization, when the lottery, generosity and dynamism of life brought a particular sperm and ovum together to cause a substantial change — the beginning of me. Thus the continuity between the adult bodily selves we are, and the embryonic bodily selves we were, is today a matter of fact. The human being as a member of his species comes into existence at fertilization and ceases to exist when he dies. This much biology can tell us.

In a recent book called *Test-Tube Babies*, one of its editors, Professor Peter Singer, says:

'When opponents of abortion say that the embryo is a living human being from conception onwards, all they can possibly mean is that the embryo is a living member of the species *homo sapiens*. This is all that can be established as a scientific fact. But is this also the sense in which every "human being" has a right to life?'[39]

Professor Singer answers the question in the negative: to be a human being does not mean to have a right to life i.e. to be recognized to have a human moral status. This is his moral

88

option. So too has been the option of the Medical Research Council, of the Ethical Committee of the RCOG, and of the British Medical Association, in the recent guide-lines they have produced concerning IVF and embryo replacement and embryo transfer. But it is an option that cannot legitimately be said to follow the Western Moral tradition 'grounded in Aristotelian thought and science'. For in this tradition, as we saw earlier, the consideration of who counts as a human being *biologically* has not been dismissed or disregarded as a sound basis for ascribing moral status. The option, of which Professor Singer is a representative, is more in accord with the utilitarian tradition. It is an option that carries with it other fundamental ones: it is necessarily a commitment to the view that not all human beings are equal; that humanity is not the universal ground of our equal status; that there are some human beings judged to be of a 'lesser kind', either because of their merely incipient organic development, or because of some other defective or damaged organic condition. The option is also a commitment to the view that 'the lesser human beings' can be of radical instrumental value for the benefit and interests of others who are better off humanly: either because they already have a central nervous system, or look human, or are born, or are adults who can reason and exercise autonomy. So the rights of the 'lesser' human beings will be subservient to the rights of the 'full' human beings. Thus, as the RCOG Report puts it, following Dr Edwards' views, when a living child may require a bone marrow transplant obtainable from an embryo, 'the rights of the 14-day embryo should be subservient to the interests of the living child' (Sec. 13.7). One would like to know with Mr David Bolt of the BMA Council what there is that is so sacrosanct about the 14 days![40]

Naturally the lesser human beings will legally become properties, and will be used and disposed of accordingly.

To opt for disregarding humanity as the basis of moral status is to depart from the egalitarian ideal that has led us to the abolition of slavery and is leading us to the abolition of any kind of apartheid; it also departs from 'the respect for life from the time of conception'[41] expected of clinicians and researchers in their tradition and their medical codes of practice; it is a departure from the non-instrumental vision of life inherent in our laws and in traditional morality, as opposed to the instrumental view of life defended by utilitarianism.

89

I cannot adhere to such a departure and the moral vision that prompts it. *The biological definition of when a new human life begins, and the moral vision recognising that human beings are not properties* and so are not to be used or exploited for any purpose whatsoever, are the firm grounds to offer for including in the human family all human beings, from conception to death, as sharing the human moral status which entitles them to protection of life. The human embryo is indeed someone in the species, a human being. The respect owed to our embryonic selves, to the earliest stages of our lives, should not be different *in kind* from the respect owed to any member of the human family for we all share in the same 'human' *kind*. This respect *minimally* implies the rights 'not to be used as a mere means to the interests of other, and not to be killed'[42].

III. Aims and means of IVF Programmes: what is permissible, what is desirable

The opening questions of my paper: what kind of respect is due to the human embryo? is the human embryo to be protected as a human being or as a property? have been answered thus: the respect due to the human embryo must not differ *in kind* from the respect due to any other human being; the human embryo must be protected as a human being, not as a property or an object of use.

In the light of these answers how are we to assess the aims and means of IVF programmes?

Let me begin by considering the ethical question raised by Dr Edwards: 'should human embryology be pursued for its own sake?' Embryology for its own sake, i.e. knowledge of embryonic life, of its structures and processes, is presently justified with principles such as these: it is desirable to learn as much as possible about human reproduction, organogenesis, and the function of genes; it is desirable to improve knowledge that will help to treat genetic and chromosomal abnormalities as well as infertility; it is desirable to do research on human embryos to learn about the human being, because such knowledge is not obtainable in any other way. Let us assume for the moment that these are all worthy aims, and that lesser aims such as some that W Walters and Professor Singer might entertain — of animal-human hybrids who "would be able to carry out unpleasant jobs and mundane tasks in the community, relieving man for more skilled occupations"[43] — are excluded.

These worthy aims are all to be carried out at the expense, use, and destruction of human lives, even if they are lives in their early beginnings. The aims justify the means. The principles that at present justify those means and aims will justify similar ones later. There is no reason why they could not be extended further, even if more developed lives are to be expended.

Most researchers will also abide by the principle that there should be no restriction on scientific research at all[44]. (The adherence of Dr D White to the principle 'plus ultra', as he put it to us in his paper, may be taken as a good illustration of this.)

On moral grounds the question 'embryology for its own sake?' must be answered in the negative. Studying and experimenting on human embryos for scientific purposes is immoral. For such experiments are never in the interest of the subject experimented upon, who is harmed, used up and destroyed: he or she is always used radically as a means, as an object of use. Thus, practices such as embryo division, freezing of embryos, observing the development of human embryos and fetuses in vitro, the generating and growing of embryos in vitro for tissue culture and transplantation, genetic manipulation of embryos, and attempts to bring about cloning, ectogenesis (i.e. the continuing development of the fetus in vitro), and hybridisation (i.e. trans-species fertilization), are all radical instrumentalisations of human lives. They are radically immoral.

Perhaps what we might all consider as acceptable in the IVF programmes is the therapeutic aim of alleviating the infertility of a married couple. Yet to achieve this good aim unethical means must also be endorsed in practice, for there must be some use or disposal of the 'spare' embryos. The spare embryos are obtained usually by the method of induced superovulation in the woman. Superovulation is seen as an advantage over spontaneous ovulation and justified on the following grounds: (i) to avoid in the woman the trauma and hazard of repeated laparoscopies for ovum recovery (such a surgical operation requires total anaesthesia); (ii) superovulation facilitates the selection of embryos before implantation; (iii) it also increases the possibility of attaining the aim of the programme: that of achieving pregnancy; for if there is a miscarriage one of the 'spare' embryos may then be implanted; (iv) if ova were always to be recovered only at the moment of spontaneous cycle ovulation, this would place a heavy burden on the team of doctors who would have to be available at that particular time[45].

It is indeed clear that generating spare embryos is the most economic procedure for attaining the general aim in view — the greater chances of pregnancy with the minimum of effort, expense, and trauma. Yet the well-being and existence of each individual life thus generated is made secondary and instrumental to the general aim. Those lives, if not required for the desired pregnancy, will be disposed of, used for experiments, or frozen until a time comes when they will again be demanded for implantation, experimentation or disposal.

We heard from Dr Edwards that the disposal or usage of embryos is justified since many other early human lives are destroyed for less worthy purposes by means of IUDs or in eugenic abortion (i.e. those abortions not done in defence of the life of the mother but for the sake of limiting the family or for the interest of society)[46]. Naturally, this raises the question of whether the direct destruction of any human life, whether by IUD, abortion, disposal or experimentation, is justified. Dr Edwards seems to imply that a society which accepts eugenic abortion has no moral grounds for prohibiting experimentation with embryos. In my opinion he is right. This whole question also shows how far and to what new fields the acceptance of abortion can reach.

A different type of justification at present being offered for the disposal of spare embryos is this: 'Knowing as we do that in the natural process large numbers of fertilised ova are lost before implantation, it is morally unconvincing to claim absolute inviolability for an organism with which nature itself is so prodigal'[47]. It is clear to us all, I think, that natural processes such as volcanic eruptions, floods, droughts and other kinds of 'natural disasters' may destroy hundreds of human lives, as well as animal lives. These are natural processes as much as the processes whereby the loss of fertilized ova naturally occur. Can these natural processes be really taken as indicative of what *we are to do*? An affirmative answer to this question would have to ignore the fact that what we intend, decide, and deliberately bring about, are *not* natural processes (and just because they are not, we are answerable for them). They cannot be measured against the natural results that nature brings about. We are moral beings. Physical nature is not. A human life, at whatever stage of its development, may come naturally to an end. No one is morally accountable for that. But if we voluntarily bring about the death of such a life, or bring it into existence with that ultimate intention, we are morally accountable for such an intention and such an action. What physical nature does is no ultimate moral standard or excuse for us. *Our direct disposal of human lives, using them as objects, instrumentalising them, or exploiting them for any purpose whatever, has no moral justification.*

What could be said of the therapeutic aim of IVF for the alleviation of infertility in a married couple when disposal or usage of spare embryos is not involved in the programme? What could be said of this 'ideal case'? Even in this case I find serious ethical objections to the programme, namely, the possible and irreparable risk of harm for the child-to-be. It is known that of the 128 children born following IVF, worldwide[48], the proportion of congenital abnormalities found in these children is no higher than in children conceived in natural circumstances. That this is the case does not resolve important ethical issues for those who want to follow the IVF programme and who are also committed to respect the inviolability of human life from its very beginning. To illustrate this, the following situation may be considered: what would be the position of a couple who, following the IVF programme for the alleviation of their infertility, find that after the fertilization of their gametes the new embryo is developing abnormally? Would replacement of the embryo in the womb for implantation be the choice, knowing that the child conceived will develop with congenital abnormalities? Would the embryo then be destroyed? Doctors now follow the policy of not implanting embryos developing abnormally. The parents cannot have the last decision in this issue, for doctors are not merely enablers in the process of IVF, but, as the RCOG Report notes, 'They are taking part in the formation of the embryo itself. That role brings a special sense of responsibility for the welfare of the child thus conceived' (Sec. 6.1).

Thus it is inherent to the procedures of the technique of IVF itself that an irreparable damage to the embryo or the child-to-be cannot be excluded. This is clearly acknowledged by Dr Edwards, when he mentions the back-up methods of monitoring abnormalities after IVF and implantation, as well as implicitly by the RCOG when they say: 'the possibility that a child born with an abnormality might in due course be able to sue its parents and the doctors, cannot be ruled out' (Sec. 10.7).

Are we justified morally in bringing about a process with such a possible risk of harm? My answer is in the negative and is

93

shared by P Ramsay [49] and L Kass[50], and, more recently, by H Teifel[51]. It is no excuse for us to say that abnormalities following IVF are similar to those following the natural process of conception. Again: nature takes care of itself, but we have to take care of *our* actions. A child brought into existence with an abnormality possibly caused as a result of his conception in vitro, where human responsibility and knowledge have directly intervened, cannot accept it in the same way as a child whose handicap is the result of a natural process where such direct human responsibility is absent. If the well-being of each individual child is the paramount interest, and not the wishes of the parents, we would not embark on such risky generation. An attitude of respect for human life — not seeking to use it as a means for the interests of others in any circumstances — must hold that just as 'a mal-formed infant has the same rights as a normal infant'[52], so a mal-developing embryo should be afforded the same respect and protection that is due to a well-developing embryo. To embark on processes where both normal embryos and defective embryos are generated and some must be discarded is immoral.

It seems clear that respect for and protection of the human embryo in accord with its human status can only in fact be guaranteed in the natural process of procreation and not in the technical IVF mode of generation, because the mal-forming embryo will never have the chance of being treated with respect: it is bound to be killed; it will not be implanted. If it were to be implanted with the knowledge that it is abnormal, it would be found practically impossible to bear the moral and legal responsibilities involved[53]. In a natural process of procreation such an embryo might or might not abort. In the IVF process it must be destroyed. In natural procreation the child is conceived and received 'for better or for worse'; in the IVF programme only conditionally — 'for better'.

Taking things as they are, knowing the present climate of opinion and the most generalised moral outlook, and being aware of the interests of researchers in this field, and the guidelines recently published, it must be accepted — although with sadness — that IVF programmes will continue, and 'embryology for its own sake' will be pursued. I say 'with sadness' because I cannot see any long-term benefit to mankind in aims and procedures which are radically objectionable on moral grounds: for they all fall short of the respect due to every human life, which should never be a mere means, or even a valuable instrument to be used for the interest and benefits of others or of society, or of science. Morality is the ground of human life. It is my view that our society as a whole, and the social practices which aim at and are directed towards the moral and total well-being and development of its members, cannot be sustained if we relinquish that basic respect for human life which I have been expressing in the principle 'no human being is a property'. 'Human being', as we have seen, applies from the beginning of his existence at conception until the end at death.

Let me permit myself to be optimistic, and allow myself to believe that IVF programmes will only develop further in the therapeutic context of alleviation of infertility. What in that case would be socially desirable? What might be recommended, not as the moral ideal, but as the lesser of two evils? I offer as proposals two principles that might guide future development of social forms of life related to human procreation:

(i) The well-being of the child must be of paramount importance; it must be recognised that the child is not a commodity, a property.

(ii) Truth — which does not exclude confidentiality — and the responsibility of all the parties involved in the process of human generation must be guaranteed by whatever means are possible.

The well-being of the child. The child must be brought into existence for his own sake, 'for better or for worse'. This is a very basic fundamental demand of all human beings, of all of us: to be loved and respected for our own sakes and not for any instrumental gains others may seek from us. A prevailing attitude in our society is that of considering the child as merely the object which satisfies a need. If desired, anything would be done to have it; if not desired it is rejected to the point of being destroyed. This attitude of regarding children as commodities will be fostered with IVF programmes. But what we cannot in fact permit is the actual *commercialisation of human generation* that such an attitude may seek. Thus, the generative procedures by which a child is brought into existence must not be commercialised. The marketing of sperm and ova, of embryos — through embryo banks — and womb leasing, etc. must all be prohibited. In the same way, if gametes are donated it must be done without any financial inducements. 'Generation' is related to 'generosity', to the 'giving' of life which is freely received and must be freely given. If the child is to be brought into existence

95

for his own sake, procedures for the selection of children on eugenic grounds, or for the moulding of their features and characters according to the interests of parties, governments or science, must all be excluded. Who are those parties to sit in judgement to determine the course of life of others? Children are not commodities designed to satisfy needs. They claim respect, care, and responsible acceptance *as equals* with us.

Truth and social responsibility. Bearing in mind the well-being of the child, I cannot subscribe to the so-called 'principle of anonymity'[54]. This is the principle governing (AID) Artificial Insemination by Donor, whereby the donor of sperm is anonymous and not made known to relatives, the parents, and the child himself. Such anonymity breeds irresponsibility. The donor, usually a medical student, is paid £7 per sample of seminal fluid and no further responsibility is *required* of him for his action[55]. Why, in AID or other forms of generation, should the child be deprived of knowing who his genetic parents are? Why are we to deprive him of the truth? Why should any action for which we are responsible — if it is a morally good action, or e.g. an action voluntarily done as an act of generosity to communicate life — be always kept anonymous? To base social relations, i.e. between doctors, donors and parents, as well as family relations, or interpersonal relations, on grounds which are not of open — though confidential — truth, and of responsibility, is to build our society on shaky foundations. Thus full documentation about donors, no financial inducement for their donations, and regulations governing both their rights and their responsibilities, must be secured.

My general recommendation, both morally and socially, is for adoption, and not for a risky technological generation ultimately involving direct destruction of human lives. We owe a living to those children already existing. We do not owe a living to those who have not yet come into existence.

My recommendation is, as well, for our continued cooperation with the commitment of our society to research and study, seeking all forms of advance for the alleviation of human suffering. These forms of advance could be addressed more directly to questions of *root causes* and of *prevention*[56] which do not involve the direct use and destruction of human lives. Indeed, genetic diseases, malformations, other forms of diseases, and human infertility — without forgetting the malnutrition and hunger that affects our world — demand of us a continuous effort to alleviate them as causes of human suffering. And whether these forms of human suffering are naturally caused, or whether they are the result of our unjust dealings with one another, they demand our commitment to their prevention and to the abolition of their real and ultimate causes. The medical and scientific aims and procedures expressing such a commitment can indeed be in accord with the respect owed to every human being, or can be re-orientated in that direction. I do not believe that 're-orientating' our means and ends in this direction implies abandoning possibilities of progress. It does indeed *not* imply bringing our research to a standstill. It means looking in other directions to discover new possibilities not previously foreseen because not previously considered. Nature, our brains, and the true generosity of our minds and hearts will not let us down in this task. In 1969 Dr Edwards said that his research with human embryos would help among other things in the discovery of the causes of Down's syndrome with a view to preventing it[57]. Professor Lejeune has contributed his views earlier in this book. In this respect Professor Lejeune's work in this particular field has been of such enormous significance and has made such a contribution. I would like to take this as an example of that commitment to research and to the progress of science and humanity which I am endorsing: tirelessly undertaken, and with the unconditional respect which is due to every human being from the beginning of his existence.

Let me finish on a note of hope. Moral issues can only be sorted out and tackled by moral means and with moral courage. There is no other solution for them than our moral strength. That key and that power is within each one of us. So, there is always hope. Recently I saw the following lines being applied to our policies of nuclear disarmament[58]; they can be applied to our present topic too. They summarise much of what I have here been trying to say:

'Point not the goal, until you plot the course,
For ends and means to man are tangled so
That different means quite different aims enforce;
Conceive the means as ends in embryo.'

NOTES

I want to express my gratitude to Dr J Finnis and to my colleagues at The Linacre Centre, Luke Gormally and Janey Milne Home, for having read this paper and for the valuable suggestions they made for its improvement. It is the byproduct of a larger piece of research and writing which I am engaged in at The Linacre Centre. At this stage of my work the views expressed there are not formally attributable to anyone other than myself.

1   The Government established a Committee of Inquiry into Human Fertilization and Embryology under the chairmanship of Mrs Mary Warnock in the autumn of 1982. The terms of reference of the inquiry were: "to consider recent and potential developments in medicine and science related to human fertilisation and embryology; to consider what policies and safeguards should be applied, including consideration of the social, ethical and legal implications of their developments and to make recommendations". The government, with a view to future legislation in this field, will then consider such recommendations.

2   The Report of the Ethics Committee of the RCOG on IVF has also adhered to some of the fundamental opinions of Dr Edwards, who presented oral evidence to the Committee. See the Report's Acknowledgements.

3   Edwards, 1969.

4   Ibid p.29. It is there said: "Can we, for example, immunise people so that fertilisation or implantation are prevented?"

5   Ibid p.28.

6   Ibid.

7   See O'Connor, 1983. This theme is developed there in relation to moral pluralism.

8   To my knowledge those who have raised and discussed this ethical question have been P Ramsey, L Kass and, more recently, H O Teifel.

9   Edwards & Purdy 1982, p.vii.

10 A reading of e.g. Edwards & Purdy, 1982, shows how many of the scientific aspects of human embryology related to IVF programmes are still unknown, and how many procedures still remain at an experimental level.

11 Edwards, 1980, p.1016.

12 Cf Report in *The Times* 'Pregnancy from frozen embryo', 3 May 1983, by T Duboudin, from Melbourne.

13 Cf Edwards & Purdy 1982, pp.219-233; also cf Steptoe & Edwards 1983.

14 Cf Edwards & Purdy 1982.

15 Ibid p.380.

16 Ibid p.384.

17 Ibid p.380.

18 Ibid p.363.

19 Cf Kass, 1981.

20 Cf Teifel, 1982.

21 Edwards' own phrase, 1971 p.89.

22 Sec. I.5.

23 Sec. III.

24 This is shown in a masterly fashion in Anscombe, 1981.

25 Turney J 'The Future in Embryo', *The Times Higher Education Supplement* 15.10.82, p.11.

26 See some of the published Evidence to the Warnock Committee, of e.g.

the Catholic bodies: *In Vitro Fertilisation: Morality and Public Policy*, by the Catholic Bishops' Joint Committee on Bio-Ethical Issues,Rathoҫlic Information Services, 1983; *Human Fertilisation — Choices for the Future*, Social Welfare Commission of the Catholic Bishops' Conference (England and Wales), Catholic Information Services, 1983; 'Submission to the Government Inquiry into Human Fertilisation and Embryology from the Joint Ethico-Medical Committee of the Catholic Union of Great Britain and the Guild of Catholic Doctors' in the *The Catholic Medical Quarterly* Vol XXXIV 2 (218) pp.75-84, May 1983.

27 See 'Evidence to the Government Enquiry into Human Fertilisation and Embryology' by the Working Party of the Royal College of General Practioners, Introduction, No. 4.

28 See Braine, 1982, in particular Appendix A.

29 This has clearly been shown by Connery, 1977.

30 See Hewson, 1975, on medieval theories of conception.

31 Aquinas, *Summa Theologica* 1a, 76, 3; Aristotle *De generatione animalium* ii, 3.73, 662-5.

32 By 'extrinsically' is meant here what Aquinas, following Aristotle, describes as the infusion of the human soul *ab extra* in the developing embryo after conception, by which the embryo is transformed into a human being. See Aristotle's *De generatione animalium* 736.b. Aquinas says e.g. 3a, 6, 4:"... in nobis ante concepitur caro quam adveniat anima rationalis" (in our case conception of the flesh preceded the coming of the rational soul); also "quia non prius est caro humana quam habeat animam rationalem" (because human flesh exists only when there is a rational soul), and "caro humana sortitur esse per animam" (human flesh receives its being through the rational soul). For Aquinas, who had the jewish-christian concept of 'creation' which Aristotle did not have, human souls are created by God at the moment of their infusion into our bodies: "... quae simul creantur dum corporibus infunduntur" (3a, 6, 3). This infusion of the human soul or its coming into the flesh *ab extra* is defended both by Aristotle and Aquinas on (i) the biological basis that there is no sufficient organisation in matter at the time of human conception to sustain a rational soul; and (ii) the activity of the rational soul shows that its nature is neither explained by nor reduced to physical activity, for the rational soul (as the agent intellect) is (a) always in act, (b) separable from matter, and (c) not conjoined to any particular bodily organ. Thus the rational soul has something of the 'divine' character. Cf Aristotle's *De Anima* and Thomas Aquinas's *Commentary on De Anima* Book III, Ch.IV. In connection with this theme see also Hewson 1975, Chapter IV 'The Twofold Spirit and Animation'.

33 François Jacob (Nobel Prize for Medicine 1965) 1973, p.313.

34 Scientists for Life 1975, p.8.

35 Lejeune et al. 1981. Cf letter to *The Times* (16 April 1983) from the zoologist Dr C B Goodhart (Gonville & Caius College, Cambridge).

36 Cf Evans & Dixler 1981, p.2325.

37 Walters & Singer 1982, p.61.

38 Ramsey 1970, p.11.

39 Walters & Singer 1982, p.60.

40 Cf *British Medical Journal* 286, 14 May 1983, p.1591.

41 *Declaration of Geneva* 1968. This requirement is even demanded of doctors by the *Declaration of Oslo* 1970, on therapeutic abortion.

42 Teifel 1982, p.3241

43 Cf J Hughes-Onslow, 'Nine months to 1984' *The Spectator* 30 April, 1983, p.16.

44 Cf Kass 1978.

45 Cf RCOG Ethics Committee Report on IVF. Sec.11.

46 Edwards 1971, p.87.

47 RCOG Ethics Committee Report on IVF, Sec.13.5.

48 Cf British Medical Association Interim Report on IVF, *British Medical Journal* 286, No.5, p.1594.

49 Kass 1978.

50 Ramsey 1980.

51 Teifel 1982.

52 British Medical Association advice on 'Severely malformed infants', *British Medical Journal* 286 (14 May 1983) p.1593.

53 Steptoe & Edwards 1983. This letter is an excellent illustration of the causes for fear that researchers have in relation to the possible implantation of abnormal embryos.

54 Cf RCOG Ethics Committee Report on IVF; also 'Maternity Alliance' Report to Warnock Committee in *Maternity Alliance Bulletin* March-April 1983, No.9.

55 Cf. Snowdon & Mitchell 1981.

56 Cf. Kass 1978.

57 Edwards 1969, p.29.

58 Cf letter to *The Times*, 'CND and Communism' from Dr Tony Weaver, 3 May 1983.

REFERENCES

Anscombe G E M
1981 'Modern Moral Philosophy' (1958), reprinted in G E M Anscombe *Ethics, Religion and Politics Collected Philosophical Papers* Vol III Blackwell, Oxford.
Aristotle
De generatione animalium
De anima
Braine D
1982 *Medical Ethics and Human Life* Palladio Press, Aberdeen.
Connery J
1977 *Abortion. The Development of the Roman Catholic Perspective* Loyola University Press, Chicago.
Evans M I & Dixler A O
1981 'Human In Vitro Fertilization' *The Journal of the American Medical Association* 245, 2324/2327.
Edwards R G
1969 'Reproduction: chance and choice' in D Paterson, Ed. *Genetic Engineering* BBC Publications
1980 *Conception in the Human Female* Academic Press, London.
Edwards R G & Purdy J M, Eds.

1982   *Human Conception in Vitro* Proceedings of the First Bourn Hall Meeting, Academic Press, London.

Edwards R G & Sharp D J

1971   'Social Values and Research in Human Embryology' *Nature* 231, 87-90

Hewson M A

1975   *Giles of Rome and the Medieval Theory of Conception* The Athlone Press, London.

Jacob F

1973   *The Logic of Life. A History of Heredity* Pantheon Books, New York (Translated from the French by B E Spillman)

Kass L

1978   *The Ethical Dimensions of In Vitro Fertilization* American Enterprise Institute for Public Policy Research, Washington D C

1981   'Implications of Prenatal Daignosis for the Human Right to Life' (1973) reprinted in Mappes T A & Zembaty J S, Eds. *Biomedical Ethics* McGraw-Hill, New York.

Lejeune J et al

1981   *The Beginning of Human Life* Law and Medicine Series of AUL Inc. Chicago.

O'Connor F

1983   'Pluralism: Justice or the Interests of the Stronger?' in *Abortion and Law* Dominican Publications, Dublin.

Ramsey P

1970   *Fabricated Man. The Ethics of Genetic Control* Yale University Press, New Haven.

1980   *On In Vitro Fertilization* Law and Medicine Series of AUL Inc. Chicago

Scientists for Life

1975   *The Position of Modern Science on the Beginning of Human Life* Sun Life, Greystone, Virginia.

Snowden R & Mitchell G D

1981   *The Artificial Family. A Consideration of Artificial Insemination by Donor* Unwin Books, London.

Steptoe P & Edwards R G

1983   'Pregnancy in an infertile patient after transfer of an embryo fertilised in vitro' Letter in *British Medical Journal* 286, 1351.

Thomas Aquinas

Summa Theologica (Prima pars q.76, 118, 119; Tertia pars q.6)

Tiefel H O

1982   'Human In Vitro Fertlisation' *The Journal of the American Medical Association* 247, 3235-3243.

Walters W A W & Singer P, Eds.

1982   *Test-Tube Babies. A guide to moral questions, present techniques and future possibilities* Oxford University Press, Auckland.

Ethical Codes, World Medical Association:

1948   *Declaration of Genea* (Amended 1968).

1964   *Declaration of Helsinki* (Amended 1975): On Biomedical Research on Human Subjects

1970   *Declaration of Oslo*: On Therapeutic Abortion.

Recent Guidelines on In Vitro Fertilization, British Medical Bodies:

1982 Medical Research Council, Statement on 'Research Related to Human Fertilisation and Embryology' *British Medical Journal* 285, 1480. (20 November 1982)

1983 Royal College of Obstetricians and Gynaecologists *Report of the RCOG Ethics Committee on In Vitro Fertilisation and Embryo Replacement or Transfer* (March).

1983 British Medical Association 'Interim Report on Human Fertilisation and Embryo Replacement and Transfer' *British Medical Journal* 286, 1594-1595 (Approved by the British Medical Association Council on 4 May 1983).

POSTSCRIPT

8
POSTSCRIPT

SIR JOHN PEEL, KCVO, DM, FRCOG, FRCP, FRCS, Hon FACOG, *past President of the Royal College of Obstetricians and Gynaecologists summed up the preceding papers, thanked the speakers and the organisers, including the Royal Society of Medicine who had hosted the meeting and moved the following resolution which was agreed by all present and was forwarded by Telex message to the Warnock Committee advising H.M. Government:*

'On behalf of the representatives attending the Quality of Life Conference held on Monday 23 May in London called by the interdenominational Order of Christian Unity we ask for assurance that control be positively provided to ensure that in vitro research respect human rights and dignity from the moment of conception (fertilization) and will avoid human vivesection'.

The O.C.U.

The Order of Christian Unity is an association composed of Christians from all denominations, united by belief in Jesus Christ as God and Saviour and together upholding His Commandments, particularly as they affect family life, education, medical ethics and the media.

The OCU works through a series of voluntary Committees corresponding to six Charter Points:

1. To promote and defend the teaching of Christianity in schools.
2. To uphold the ideal of chastity outside and fidelity inside marriage.
3. To uphold marriage as a permanent partnership and oppose unrestricted divorce.
4. To campaign for truth and improve the Christian content of the mass media.
5. To oppose unrestricted abortion.
6. To oppose euthanasia and support alternative caring services.

These Committees are made up of Christians with a particular concern for the well-being of the family in their field of expertise. The OCU publishes a regular newsletter "Love and Life" and also organises the annual *Sanctity of Life Night of Prayer*. It is actively seeking new members from all Christian denominations who should write in for further information from:

Order of Christian Unity
Christian Unity House
58 Hanover Gardens
London
SE11 5TN